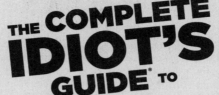

THE **COMPLETE IDIOT'S GUIDE** TO

Quick Total Body Workouts

by Tom Seabourne, Ph.D.

ALPHA

A member of Penguin Group (USA) Inc.

ALPHA BOOKS

Published by the Penguin Group

Penguin Group (USA) Inc., 375 Hudson Street, New York, New York 10014, USA • Penguin Group (Canada), 90 Eglinton Avenue East, Suite 700, Toronto, Ontario M4P 2Y3, Canada (a division of Pearson Penguin Canada Inc.) • Penguin Books Ltd., 80 Strand, London WC2R 0RL, England • Penguin Ireland, 25 St. Stephen's Green, Dublin 2, Ireland (a division of Penguin Books Ltd.) • Penguin Group (Australia), 250 Camberwell Road, Camberwell, Victoria 3124, Australia (a division of Pearson Australia Group Pty. Ltd.) • Penguin Books India Pvt. Ltd., 11 Community Centre, Panchsheel Park, New Delhi—110 017, India • Penguin Group (NZ), 67 Apollo Drive, Rosedale, North Shore, Auckland 1311, New Zealand (a division of Pearson New Zealand Ltd.) • Penguin Books (South Africa) (Pty.) Ltd., 24 Sturdee Avenue, Rosebank, Johannesburg 2196, South Africa • Penguin Books Ltd., Registered Offices: 80 Strand, London WC2R 0RL, England

First edition originally published as *The Pocket Idiot's Guide to a Great Upper Body*, *The Pocket Idiot's Guide to Great Abs*, and *The Pocket Idiot's Guide to Great Buns & Thighs*

Copyright © 2012 by Penguin Group

International Standard Book Number: 978-1-61564-158-1
Library of Congress Catalog Card Number: 2011912285

14 13 12   8 7 6 5 4 3 2 1

Interpretation of the printing code: The rightmost number of the first series of numbers is the year of the book's printing; the rightmost number of the second series of numbers is the number of the book's printing. For example, a printing code of 12-1 shows that the first printing occurred in 2012.

Printed in the United States of America

Note: This publication contains the opinions and ideas of its author. It is intended to provide helpful and informative material on the subject matter covered. It is sold with the understanding that the author and publisher are not engaged in rendering professional services in the book. If the reader requires personal assistance or advice, a competent professional should be consulted.

The author and publisher specifically disclaim any responsibility for any liability, loss, or risk, personal or otherwise, which is incurred as a consequence, directly or indirectly, of the use and application of any of the contents of this book.

Most Alpha books are available at special quantity discounts for bulk purchases for sales promotions, premiums, fundraising, or educational use. Special books, or book excerpts, can also be created to fit specific needs.

For details, write: Special Markets, Alpha Books, 375 Hudson Street, New York, NY 10014.

Publisher: *Marie Butler-Knight*
Associate Publisher/Acquiring Editor: *Mike Sanders*
Executive Managing Editor: *Billy Fields*
Development Editor: *Susan Zingraf*
Senior Production Editor: *Kayla Dugger*
Copy Editor: *Tricia Liebig*

Cover Designer: *Kurt Owens*
Book Designers: *William Thomas, Rebecca Batchelor*
Indexer: *Celia McCoy*
Layout: *Brian Massey*
Proofreader: *John Etchison*

ALWAYS LEARNING   PEARSON

This book is dedicated to my father, who will always be my inspiration; to my wife, Danese; and to Jeff Tuller, Mindy Mylrea, and the thousands of fitness professionals around the world trying to make a difference.

Contents

Introduction

It's hard to take your eyes off a well-developed body. A ripped upper body, chiseled abs, and a firm butt and thighs is quite a package, and it's a package that can and will be yours with the help of this book. All you need are three ingredients explained here: the motivation to work out, an eating plan that fuels muscles and starves fat, and exercises that sculpt your body.

Start your mind-body journey to define your arms, lose your gut, and lift your butt, just to name some of what you can accomplish with the information in this book. You have the desire because you picked up this book; now make the commitment. In a week, you will notice muscles that you didn't know existed. And when you start to see results in the mirror, like a flatter tummy and slimmer hips, you'll be hooked.

The purpose of this book is not to turn you into an exercise fanatic or a health-food nut. There is no need to exercise for hours a day or eat perfectly all the time. Exercise a little each day, eat right most of the time, and stay consistent with it, and you're on your way to a healthy, toned, and beautiful body.

How This Book Is Organized

This book is divided into four parts:

Part 1, Keys to Success, covers the overall scope of your workout program. It discusses how to get your mind set up to meet your goals for your body, the proper techniques for successful workouts, an eating program that will help you achieve long-term success, and how to put everything together to develop and maintain the body you've always dreamed of.

Part 2, Upper Body, provides exercises that will cut and define the muscles in your chest, back, shoulders, and arms. You will learn upper-body workouts you can do at the gym, at home, even at the office, as well as stretches to keep you flexible and feeling good.

Part 3, Abdominals, shows you how to work the four muscle groups in your abdomen—your internal and external obliques, your six-pack, and underneath it all your transverse abdominis. Stretches and exercises you can perform at home, the gym, and the office will help you firm up your stomach and love handles.

Part 4, Buns and Thighs, explores exercises you can do at home, the gym, and the office to tone and tighten the muscles in your legs, thighs, and butt—including hamstrings, glutes, and hips. You'll also learn stretches for the buns, thighs, and legs to help maximize your workouts.

Extras

In this book, you will find sidebars that are tidbits of important and useful information to help you along the way.

> **BET YOU DIDN'T KNOW**
>
> Common myths and misconceptions concerning diet and exercise, and what the truths really are.

> **GET IT RIGHT**
>
> Cautionary warnings to be sure you're doing your exercises right.

> **IN OTHER WORDS**
>
> Explanations of the anatomy of different muscles and of technical or unusual terms.

> **YOUR PERSONAL TRAINER**
>
> Quick tips about how to do your exercises correctly and keep your form perfect.

Acknowledgments

I want to thank the photographer, Ron Barker, and our fabulous models, Brittany Scott and Brandon Sears. My wife Danese, and five beautiful children Alaina, Grant, Laura, Susanna, and Julia, who are always finding ways to make workouts fun. And finally my brother, Rick, my sister, Barb, and my mother, Ann.

Trademarks

All terms mentioned in this book that are known to be or are suspected of being trademarks or service marks have been appropriately capitalized. Alpha Books and Penguin Group (USA) Inc. cannot attest to the accuracy of this information. Use of a term in this book should not be regarded as affecting the validity of any trademark or service mark.

Keys to Success

This part covers the overall scope of your workout program. It discusses how to get your mind set up to meet your goals for your body, the proper techniques for successful workouts, an eating program that will help you achieve long-term success, and how to put everything together to develop and maintain the body you've always dreamed of.

Your Training Mindset

In This Chapter

- Setting your goals
- Keeping from quitting
- Managing distractions and injuries
- Picturing your new body

Congratulations! Purchasing this book is an important step in getting a toned and sculpted body. Choose your goal—having a well-developed chest, or just being able to wear a sleeveless tee shirt; losing your love handles or getting a six-pack; lifting your buns or slimming your hips. Setting quick goals will keep you pumped up for the long haul. Don't compare your progress to others; it takes them just as long as it takes you.

Take a minute and think about what you will look like in a bathing suit after a couple months of working out. Create a detailed mental picture of your defined upper, mid, and lower body. Find a picture of a person you admire or would like to look like with your same body structure to motivate you.

Brain Training Is Key

A quick examination of how your goals and desires fit your personality can go a long way toward helping you stay with your exercise program. You may prefer to work out at home, in the office, in a gym, or all of the above. Your personality may lead you to a strict regimen, or cross-training in a variety of exercises.

Don't just start working out. Get on a program you believe in. This will increase your motivation and provide you with the confidence to stick with your workout to deliver the results you desire.

Although you may have given up on working out in the past, this program is doable. You don't have to pick one form of exercise and plod through it for the rest of your life. Any exercise that gets you off the couch is fine.

Schedule Your Workout to Fit

Be honest. In the past, when you missed workouts or quit programs, it was partly because you were lazy. This program will help you figure out what works for you when it comes to staying motivated for longer than a week or two.

Schedule your meals and workout into your day. The best time to work out is whenever it consistently fits into your schedule. Working out in the morning is a great way to start your day. It's an energizing way to stimulate your metabolism, and there is less chance that your workout will be interrupted.

Scheduling your workout for later in the evening may be a disaster. Putting off your training until after work or dinner usually means that it won't get done. Before you know it, you will feel sleepy and it's bedtime.

Schedule your workout for a set exact time on each workout day. Be faithful to this schedule no matter what.

To get started, your favorite 30-minute easy daily activity plus a couple days of toning and stretching is all you need. Keep your workouts balanced and progressing. This will keep you motivated.

Fifty percent of those who begin an exercise program quit within the first six months because of lack of time, injury, negative emotions, poor social support, or low motivation. You can be in the successful 50 percent that faces these adversities and overcomes them.

Finding the Workout That Works

A combination of your eating program and isolation training is your blueprint for a tight, toned body. But you have to get started. First thing tomorrow morning, schedule your workout.

But be careful—an overzealous training schedule might be the last thing you need. Start slow and progress gradually. Choose activities you love. People who stick with their workout programs are not more disciplined than you. They have simply found a program that they look forward to doing.

Create workouts that aren't workouts. Any easy activity counts toward your exercise time. Moving around feels good and getting up and out the door gives you a break from your normal routine.

The back of your arms won't stop waving after one workout, your stomach won't be a rock, and your thighs will still jiggle, but you will feel so much better about yourself. Your energy level will increase and you will catch yourself glancing in the mirror to check yourself out. Use the photos in this book to motivate your training. Give yourself a reasonable amount of time to notice results.

Your body doesn't know whether you are walking or skating. Your muscles will firm up whether you use free weights or exercise bands. If you hate the thought of "working" out, go out and play with your kids or have fun with a sport. Push your kids on swings, or play volleyball or tennis. Different activities keep your exercise program balanced. Try new things to keep your fitness moving forward. Use muscles you haven't used before. Challenge your coordination with one-legged exercises. Try playing a game of catch with your other hand.

Most people start working out too hard or not hard enough. If you can only endure for five minutes, so be it. Add 2 minutes a week until you are training for 30 minutes. You don't have to work out at your target heart rate five days a week and eat like a health nut. Re-evaluate your goals so that your exercise is specific to what you really want.

If you don't have much time to work out, break up your program into manageable parts. A full half hour may be out of the question, so separate your workout into three 10-minute segments.

Keeping a log of your workouts can help prevent overtraining or undertraining. Writing down how long you walked or how much weight you lifted is objective evidence that you are making progress.

Integrating Workouts and Life

Make your eating program and workouts a habit. Do not miss any meals or workouts for your first month. Clear your schedule so there are no conflicts.

If you dread exercise and eating properly, tell yourself you can quit after a month. Reward yourself after each successful day of eating and exercise with massages, manicures, or clothing. Create short- and long-term goals as well for motivational purposes.

After you have been working out for a while, instead of choosing the best "calorie burner," ask your body how the new workout makes you feel.

During your easy-activity workouts, let your mind wander. Your most creative ideas will come to you when you're doing a repetitive activity that doesn't require your full concentration. But don't set out to cure cancer. Use your easy-activity time to answer less-pressing questions so your workouts don't become work.

You may be the type of person who needs to get pumped up before you work out. But being too jazzed causes you to lose focus. And if you are too relaxed, you may catch yourself reclining on the couch. Get pumped up, but not too much. Your mind affects your workout. Use music, TV, or whatever it takes to tie those shoes and get moving.

Eating rituals are important, too. Schedule meals in advance and sit down to all of your meals. Be consistent. Discipline is a skill that improves with practice. It is better to be consistent and steady than to be perfect for a week and then quit.

GET IT RIGHT

You should feel energized and revitalized after your workout. If you feel sluggish and tired, you did too much.

You don't have to join a gym, but it sure helps. Sign up for a long-term membership so that you will be wasting your hard-earned money if you don't go. You will make new friends at the gym. Choose a friend as a training partner. Meet your partner at a specific time to work out. Training with like-minded people is motivating, a bit of healthy competition is fun, and a commitment with a workout partner is difficult to break, too!

YOUR PERSONAL TRAINER

Partner training is great for your motivation. Choose a reliable partner.

Pushing Through the Burn

Stay cool no matter what. If something goes wrong during your workout, note it, adjust, and then go on. If you don't get to all of your exercises, tell yourself you will get to them next time.

Even your best-laid plans may go awry. A phone call five minutes before your workout or an unexpected trip out of town can ruin your schedule. Have a backup plan. Reschedule your activity or take an exercise band in your suitcase for your out-of-town workouts.

Change negative feelings and thoughts that distract you from your goal. Mentally prepare for an unexpected event. If the phone rings during your home workout, let the answering machine pick it up. Make fitness a priority in your life, and you will have a firm and tight upper body before you know it.

If you strain a muscle, see your physician and ask if there is a way to work around the problem. Be open to doing different activities outside of your usual regimen.

BET YOU DIDN'T KNOW

If you strain a muscle in your arm or leg, don't forget about the other 75 percent of your body that is looking forward to your workout.

No matter your intentions, it's not *if* you miss a workout, it's *when*. You are not perfect in other areas of your life, and your workouts won't be perfect, either. Obsessing about exercise is worse than not exercising at all. If you feel as if you can't miss a day, you may be setting yourself up for an overuse injury. Your muscles need to rest and rejuvenate at least one day each week; your mind needs a day off, too. A day off may be just what you need to attack your workout the next day. Giving yourself a mental break prevents burnout and makes you more likely to stick to your long-term exercise program.

IN OTHER WORDS

Abstinence violation is psycho-babble that means when you miss a day of your workout or eating program, you decide to give up and throw in the towel.

Plan for lapses and relapses. Too many people fall off the wagon and then give up. Lapses are part of this program. Cheating on meals and an occasional week off from exercise are not only acceptable, they're required. Skip a workout on purpose to prove to yourself that falling off the wagon is no big deal. The next day, get right back on the wagon.

Add a Ritual or Consistent Routine

Create your own rituals in your workouts. For instance, before bicep curls, set your feet, bring your elbows in close, bring your shoulders back, put your chest out, take a deep breath, and begin your first rep.

Don't rush through your workout. How many times have you seen gym rats (not you, of course) using their backs to swing the weights up, instead of using good form? They strain their muscles so bad they can't work out for a month.

Try this strategy to work the proper muscles and stay safe: Begin by sitting with perfect posture. Squeeze your hands into fists; relax. Bring your shoulders toward your ears; relax. Press your heels into the floor; relax. Press your lower back into the chair; relax.

This teaches you to be aware of your muscles while you are training them. Then, when you are doing your exercises, you will notice if you are unnecessarily straining other muscles.

Visualize Your New Body

You want to have firm arms, a streamlined back, a six-pack stomach, and a butt that turns heads. Imagine what you will look like after a month on the program. If you think you are too tired to work out, begin your warm-up. If you still feel tired, go for an easy stroll instead of doing your full-blown power walk.

Picture the training it will take to look good in your swimsuit. When you visualize yourself training, nervous impulses are sent down pathways to stimulate muscle fibers. So you're actually getting a workout just thinking about your well-defined upper body.

Imagine performing the bench press. Pretend you are lying on your back on the bench. Pull your shoulder blades together, your feet firmly planted on the floor, and grab the steel bar. Feel your chest muscles flexing as you take the bar off of the rack and lower it toward your chest. Congratulations. You actually created a mind-to-muscle connection.

Watch a mental movie of yourself training. All elite athletes do this. Seeing your workout before you do it is not hocus-pocus; it makes your workouts easier and more effective. Imagine you are in the cafeteria line. What foods will you choose?

Place your right hand on your left upper arm. Feel the definition. Imagine yourself doing a bicep curl. Feel the imaginary flexing of your arm muscles. The more you practice in your head, the more ripped and toned your arms will become. Do the same for your abs and lower body.

Daydream about your goals and you'll get them. Self-talk such as "My arms are becoming defined," "My hips are getting slimmer," or "My abs are getting tighter" raises your enthusiasm. Use your sense of humor every chance you get. Keep your mind on your workout. Use emotions to pump up or relax. Feel strong and know that your body can handle the physical effort. Remain confident no matter what.

The Least You Need to Know

- Set specific and quick goals for your exercise program.
- Joining a gym and finding a workout partner are helpful in reaching your workout goals.
- Missing workouts will happen, but it doesn't have to throw off your whole routine and goals.
- Visualize the body you want and the training it will take to achieve it.

Proper Techniques

In This Chapter

- Realizing the importance of good form
- Learning how resistance training works
- Putting variety in your sets
- Understanding rest

When working your muscles, proper form and technique is as important as doing the exercises themselves. Poor form or technique is a recipe for muscle strain, soreness, and injury. This chapter explains proper form and technique when exercising your muscle groups.

Form

All exercises should be performed in a controlled manner and in a range of motion that is comfortable. Keep your form perfect and maintain normal breathing.

Maintain Perfect Posture

Keep your stomach in; relax your neck; keep your back flat (don't arch). Draw your navel in toward your spine by contracting your lower abs. Do this before and during all of your exercises.

Focus on a specific part of your body. For example, to train your chest, think about pushing away from your body. Relax the remainder of your body so a higher percentage of force is exerted behind the specific muscle group you are working.

Place the palm of your hand just below your navel. Pooch your stomach out as if attempting to pose for the "before" picture on an infomercial. Then use your lower-stomach muscles to slowly squeeze your lower abs toward your spine and hold for three seconds. Relax for a few seconds and try it again. Do this exercise for a few reps. Then, whenever you're performing exercises, remember to flex these muscles before and during all of your reps.

Weight or Reps Don't Dictate Form

Move smoothly into each repetition with a controlled and yet 100 percent energized effort, keeping the rest of your body relaxed.

Move through a full range of motion on each of your upper-body exercises. Ease into your workout. Start with some easy repetitions, and then gradually increase the intensity. Breathe normally during an exercise; however, if you are exerting, exhale during the contraction. Inhale on your short rests between each contraction.

Balance is important for symmetrical development of your muscles. An unbalanced workout program can lead to a difference in strength between your arms or legs or chest and back. When this happens, you are more susceptible to injuries.

Muscle groups that oppose each other need to be balanced. Development between each side and the fronts and backs should be balanced. Fortunately, this program has built-in exercises so that you will be training all of your muscle groups.

Speed

Take your time on each repetition. The slower you move, the less momentum, and the more work your muscles are accomplishing. You should be able to stop at any point during your rep.

Three Seconds Both Directions

During each repetition of your workout, there are two different phases. One is called the *positive* or "up" phase of the repetition. The second is the *negative* or "down" phase of the repetition. It is important to come down slowly on the negative phase. Moving slowly on the negative phase will speed your progress to chisel that new body.

Go Slow

Don't worry about how much weight or how many reps you can do. Instead, think about the quality of your movement. If you are too fatigued to do the negative portion of the rep with perfect control, then you have done enough reps for that exercise.

Your muscles will respond very well when you are using good form at a controlled speed. Cheating on your reps leads to injury. Don't try to keep up with someone else. Work at your own pace.

Resistance

Resistance training tones your muscles. Use dumbbells, bands, or your own body weight to challenge your different muscle groups. Pushing and pulling are forms of resistance, too.

Training your body with resistance increases your lean muscle mass. The more lean muscle you have, the more calories your body burns. There is no better way to contour and streamline your body than by using resistance. You cannot spot-lose body fat, but you can tone your muscles.

Your metabolism may be defined as how many calories your body uses, even while sleeping, breathing, or reading this book. Muscle makes up about 25 percent of your metabolic rate. Muscle tissue burns more calories than fat tissue, with each pound burning about 50 calories a day. Each pound of fat only burns about 2 calories a day.

A major factor behind losing your metabolism is muscle loss. After age 25 you lose about a half-pound of muscle each year. If you don't start toning, you will lose 5 pounds of muscle and replace it with about 15 pounds of fat every decade. It's no wonder that your friends who eat the same now as they did in high school are 30 pounds overweight. Resistance training helps shrink flab. The muscle tissue firms up to speed your sluggish metabolism. Muscle is toned and more compact than fat.

Your muscles will tone and tighten in response to repetitive exercise against progressively increased resistance. As your muscles adapt to a given weight, that weight must be gradually increased to stimulate further improvement. The key to strength and muscle tone is the overload principle. Overloading involves applying a greater-than-normal stress to your upper-body muscles. The overload may be increased weight, reps, sets, or less rest between sets. Exercises that do not overload your muscles have little benefit.

Your body won't get muscle-bound from resistance training. Women are especially concerned that they will develop huge arms or thighs. Because females don't have high levels of testosterone, they won't get big and bulky if they train the right way. Even swimsuit models lift weights.

IN OTHER WORDS

Isometric exercise is where your muscles flex, but there is no movement. Isotonic exercise takes your muscles through a full range of motion. A full range of motion is best to develop the entire muscle.

The intensity of your training is important to your progress. Intensity depends on how many reps and sets you do, how much resistance you use, and how much rest you take between sets.

Duration is how long it takes for you to complete your workout. Your workout should not take more than an hour. Ideally, each session should be completed within 45 minutes. Training too long may have a detrimental effect on your adherence.

Frequency is how often you train your muscle group, such as two times per week. The rest between workouts allows your muscles time to recover from the stress of the workout and for them to become toned and stronger.

Evaluate yourself. If your muscle group is feeling stronger and more toned and you're not gaining additional body fat, you are doing everything right.

At first, your body weight is enough resistance. Soon your muscles will adapt and you may add resistance using bands, free weights, or machine weights. Your goal will be to do 10 reps with about 75 percent of the maximum resistance you can handle.

When you begin to use resistance, start with a very light weight. Be sure you can perform 10 repetitions with perfect form before advancing to a heavier weight. Gradually add weight. Do not increase your resistance more than 5 percent in a single workout.

If you do not have adjustable bands or plates, perform more repetitions at your previous intensity. Most equipment has 10-pound weight increments.

Sets

At first, perform only 1 set of each exercise. In addition to being time efficient, single-set training is almost as effective as multiple-set training.

Do one exercise for each muscle in every muscle group. Always work your larger muscles before your smaller ones. For example, it makes no sense to do a set of close grip push-ups before a set of bench presses. If you fatigue the backs of your arms by doing the close grip push-ups, you won't have enough strength to perform well on the bench press. Both of these exercises target the backs of the arm muscles. The muscles in the backs of your arms become the weak link in the chain.

Instead, do a set of bench presses followed by a set of close grip push-ups. In this case, your chest muscles won't fatigue before the backs of your arms do.

Do One to Three Sets

After you have trained for a few months, your muscle groups can handle more than 1 set of a particular exercise. Do up to 3 sets of each exercise.

If you have a break in form, stop immediately. A break in form signals that you've worked your muscles enough. Losing your form means you can't finish your reps without changing your body position.

Whether you've done 1 set or 3 sets, after you've groaned out that wobbly rep, you're done. Pay attention to your form rep by rep.

Consecutively or Circuits

If one of your goals is to lose body fat, move quickly from one exercise to the next. Keep charts to record how you are advancing in each of your muscle groups. Write down how many sets and reps, how much resistance you are using, and how much rest you take between sets. As you increase the resistance and the number of repetitions, your muscles will respond.

When you are ready for an additional challenge, do a circuit. Perform 1 set of each exercise without rest. This burns more calories than straight sets of exercises.

Circuit training also forces your cardiovascular system to work overtime. Without resting between sets, you increase the amount of time you spend toning your body compared with the amount of time you spend resting. This increases the metabolic demand of the workout while maintaining your body strength.

Pulsing through your exercises is another way to add intensity. The principle behind pulsing is that instead of doing full-range-of-motion exercises, you just stay at your mid-range and do partial reps. Pulsing preps your body for using more resistance because it allows you to overload the parts of your muscles that are strongest, without being limited by the part of the movement where you're weakest.

Do 3 sets of 10 pulsing repetitions, resting one minute between each set. Follow that up with a regular set of 10 full-range-of-motion exercises.

Choose an exercise that you have difficulty doing for a single rep. Perform 10 sets of 1 repetition, resting 30 seconds between each set.

This is a fabulous workout because you end up performing 10 repetitions of an exercise you normally can only do for 1 or 2 reps. This program requires you to recruit more total muscle fibers than usual.

Reverse your sets and reps. Take your current set and rep scheme and reverse it. Because you normally do 3 sets of 10 reps, try 10 sets of 3 reps. Because you're stopping at 3 reps instead of 10, rest 10 seconds or less between sets. Reversing your sets and reps allows you to do the same number of total repetitions, but increases the average amount of force your muscles apply during the exercise.

Another way to change your program is to cut your workout in half. Believe it or not, you may be overtraining your muscles. By reducing the demand on them, you'll allow them to recover. Another option would be to take a week off. When you come back stronger after this break, you'll know you were overtraining.

Giant sets consist of performing three different exercises for your muscles consecutively. Set one is performed, directly followed by a set of the second and third exercise. There is minimal rest between the exercises, but rest between sets is about one minute.

A superset is performing two different exercises for two opposing muscle groups consecutively. Set one for the fronts of your arms or legs is performed, directly followed by a set for the backs. There is minimal rest in between the exercises. For example, do a set of reverse curls followed by a set of dips.

Negatives are flexing your body muscles as they lengthen. These are performed by completing a set and then having a training partner help you with the up phase of your exercise.

After you have completed a set of 10 repetitions, you should be using enough weight so that your muscles are depleted and cannot perform another rep with perfect form. Your muscles are so fatigued that you need help from your training partner to complete the up phase of any additional reps. Let your partner aid you in the up phase, then perform the negative portion of the exercise on your own with your partner's guidance.

Reps

Strength gains are not only achieved by increasing the amount of resistance you are using. Increasing the number of repetitions you perform will make your muscles stronger. If you increase the number of repetitions you can perform with good form, you have increased your strength and most likely your muscle tone as well.

Ten Repetitions Is Enough

Doing hundreds of repetitions is kind of like chewing gum. You don't get a trimmed, toned jaw if you chew a lot of gum. Also, if you could do hundreds of reps with perfect form, you'd be overdue for adding resistance. Ten reps of each exercise is enough, and when those get easy, add resistance.

When you train your muscles, you damage your muscle fibers. After your workout, your body begins to repair those fibers, a process that requires calories.

Added resistance to your body training requires you to use more muscle fibers. You'll increase the number of fibers that are damaged and burn more calories.

Fewer Reps for Strength

Do 10 repetitions for each exercise. Increase the weight and do fewer reps (6 to 8) if your goal is to gain strength in your muscles. Add enough weight to challenge your muscles but not enough to compromise your form.

More Reps for Endurance

Complete 10 to 12 repetitions with 75 percent of your maximum resistance if your goal is muscular endurance. Ten reps is a good compromise for both absolute strength and muscular endurance.

Rest

Training your muscle groups two days a week each is more than enough. Figure out which days will work best in your busy schedule. Spread your days out to get enough rest between your workouts.

Depending on how many days a week you want to work out, you may split up your routine in a variety of ways. For example, here is a six-day split routine for the upper body:

- Monday: Chest and triceps
- Tuesday: Back, biceps, and shoulders
- Wednesday: Legs and abs
- Thursday: Follow Monday routine
- Friday: Follow Tuesday routine
- Saturday: Follow Wednesday routine

You can apply this same idea to your mid- and lower-body muscle groups. There are certainly no absolutes when it comes to splitting up your routine. If you are making progress, stick with your program. If you plateau, change things up to shock your muscles.

YOUR PERSONAL TRAINER

There are no good or bad exercises, but some are better than others. Choose those that tone your body without creating aches and pains.

Less Than a Minute

Rest no longer than a minute between sets of any exercise. Do not dawdle between exercises. If you rest too long, you may lose "the pump" and decide to call it a day. Rest a minute between sets of your workouts. Short, frequent rest periods during a workout are important so that your muscles don't burn out too early in your program.

During your rest period, blood delivers oxygen and energy to your muscles and carries away waste products.

Long and Short Rests

Rest longer on heavy sets and shorter on light sets. Keep track of how much time you rest between sets in your workout. As your conditioning improves, perform the same total number of sets and reps, but lessen your rest periods to a maximum of 45 seconds. This requires your muscles to recover faster between sets and increases your results.

The harder the set, the more rest you need. One way to maximize your time is to superset your exercises, and take less rest between sets.

Two to Three Days In Between

Your muscles should be given 48 to 72 hours of rest before attacking them again. Your muscles firm up between training days. However, too much rest between workouts can hurt your progress. In as little as 96 hours, the benefits of your hard work can begin to disappear.

The Least You Need to Know

- Slow your speed to ensure your muscles are doing the work as opposed to momentum.
- Strength is gained from increasing resistance and repetitions.
- Circuit training adds more cardiovascular exercise to your workout.
- Rest two or three days between workouts of the same muscle group.

Eating Well

In This Chapter

- How to choose the right carbs
- Why a little fat and lots of water are so important
- Why a treat doesn't have to mean total failure
- How to feed muscle and starve fat

You may have tried one diet after another with no long-term success. Perhaps you tried a low- or no-carbohydrate diet and noticed a rapid weight loss, only to gain it all back in water weight a few short weeks later. Or perhaps those same foods you abandoned when you started your diet were the ones you binged on and couldn't resist any longer, and you fell off the wagon. You may have thought it was your fault that you couldn't resist the cravings and blamed your lack of willpower. But you didn't fail. Your diet failed.

To slim down the flab on the backs of your arms, get rid of stubborn abdominal fat, and reduce cellulite in your buns and thighs, you have to eat right. The layer of fat between your skin and muscles is the problem. A good eating program, as discussed in this chapter, is the solution.

Your New Food Lifestyle

Rather than viewing changes in your eating as "going on a diet," see it as a lifestyle change with modifications to your existing nutrition and foods that will make the change easier to maintain.

Keep a food journal to keep track of your nutritional and caloric intake. Simply write down the foods you eat for a week. Keep track of when, what, and why you ate. Did you eat because you were hungry, bored, tired, or nervous? You don't have to keep a diary forever, but it is one of the best tools to get you the body you want. It may be tedious at first, but it requires you to pay attention to everything you eat.

By keeping a food journal, you can also see what your body is responding to in a positive way or what is hindering you in your progress. You may find that you are not getting enough of one thing and too much of another.

BET YOU DIDN'T KNOW

Any diet that restricts a certain food group won't work in the long term. Short-term diets yield short-term results.

Healthy eating requires discipline, motivation, planning, and commitment. Also, it's important to get enough fresh air and sleep and to minimize stress—all of which contribute to poor eating habits when you're not getting enough of them.

How Food Works

When you do not eat enough, your body naturally slows its energy expenditure. Whether it is a famine or just a long time between feedings, your body has a protective mechanism so you do not need to eat as much food during lean times. That worked great during caveman days. Unfortunately, in times of plenty, nature's protective energy conservation translates into a coating of fat surrounding your upper body, abs, buns, and thighs.

The Carbs That Count

At first you might lose weight on a low-carb diet, but the loss of muscle and resulting metabolic slowdown causes you to regain weight. These diets also restrict fruits, vegetables, and whole grains, making them tough to stay on.

> **BET YOU DIDN'T KNOW**
>
> You lose weight quickly on a low-carb diet, but what the scale doesn't tell you is that most of your weight loss is water and muscle.

The truth is carbs aren't good for you—*they're fantastic!* You just have to make sure you're eating the right kind of carbs. There are calorically dense (processed) carbs and nutrient-dense carbs. Calorically dense carbs are man-made, refined, and contain a lot of calories per serving, such as pasta, bagels, and boxed cereals. Nutrient-dense carbohydrates energize your muscles for the long haul. These include fruits, veggies, and whole grains. They are packed with vitamins, minerals, and fiber. Most fruits and veggies contain fewer calories than processed carbs and give you the energy you need without adding fat to your physique. The proof? There has never been a single case of someone getting fat by eating apples and oranges.

Colorful veggies such as sweet potatoes, tomatoes, kale, spinach, broccoli, peppers, and carrots are vitamin arsenals that you cannot get enough of. The deeper and darker the color, the better for your body. So eat them as often as possible.

Fruits, veggies, and whole grains provide you with quick energy to power your workouts. They also contain fiber and other compounds that are essential to uncovering your muscles. Nutrient-dense carbs are your muscles' best source of energy—they're rocket fuel for your muscles. Think of your diet as feeding your muscle and starving your fat. Eat and drink just enough to satisfy.

The bottom line is carbs aren't the problem, too many calories are. Don't eat more calories than you use and your body won't turn to mush. If you eat more than you burn, regardless of the source of those calories (carbohydrates, proteins, or fats), your flab will grow.

If you're a marathon runner or ultra-distance cyclist, you burn up a lot of extra calories, so a high-calorie diet is appropriate. But if you work a desk job and don't have the time to run, bike, or swim several hours a day burning all those calories, you should try to only eat nutrient-dense carbs.

Protein Power

Besides nutrient-dense carbs, another major staple in your diet is lean protein. Eat a serving of protein about the size of a deck of cards at each meal. Protein is muscle-building fuel as long as you eat enough carbs with it. If you eat enough nutrient-dense carbs, then it allows protein to do its job. If you eat too few carbs, the protein you eat has no choice but to be used for energy.

Whether you get your protein from beef, pork, chicken, or turkey, go for the leaner cuts. If you are a vegetarian, eat low-fat dairy, tofu, and lots of beans and legumes.

Even the leanest animal protein contains fat, and eating too much saturated fat is not heart-healthy. The solution is to eat the right kind of fat. Garnish your meat, fruits, and veggies with healthy omega-3 monounsaturated and unsaturated fats. Nuts, seeds, and peanut butter are also tasty, fat-chiseling essential fats. Eat fish several days a week. Fish is rich in omega-3 fat and protein.

> **YOUR PERSONAL TRAINER**
>
> Diet sodas don't satisfy a thirst craving the way water can. And if you miss the potato chip crunch, choose cauliflower, broccoli, peppers, carrots, or celery.

Protein slow-releases carbs so that you feel full longer. This nourishes your muscles and decreases fat stores surrounding the hard-earned muscles of your upper body. Protein is also the foundation for your muscle. Besides water and nutrient-dense carbs, protein is the most important macro-nutrient in your body-sculpting program.

Friendly Fats

Carbs and protein have 4 calories per gram. That doesn't mean much until you find out that fat has 9 calories per gram. Combine a serving of protein and a serving of carbs and it doesn't equal one serving of fat.

Fat has more than twice the calories as protein or carbs, but fat is not your enemy. You just need to eat the right kind of fat.

Fat is important in your diet because it makes you feel full. You may eat all of the carbs in the house, but until you eat a morsel containing some fat, you may not be satisfied.

Fat disperses flavors across your tongue. This gives your taste buds a chance to experience a wide range of flavors (sweet, sour, spicy) to create a feeling of satiety or satisfaction.

Drizzle a tablespoon of olive oil, flaxseed oil, or canola oil into your eating program. Eat omega-3 fatty acids, which are found in fish, whenever you can.

Omega-3 fatty acids from fish, flaxseed oil, and canola oil improve nerve conduction, lubricate your joints and skin, and have been touted as the next miracle anti-aging agent.

YOUR PERSONAL TRAINER

Grab a handful of seeds or nuts. Peanut butter on whole wheat is also a great source of essential fat.

Lots of Water

Water is a very important part of a healthy diet. You need water as a coolant, to digest and absorb food, transport nutrients, build and rebuild cells, remove waste products, and enhance circulation.

Most people walk around dehydrated and don't even realize it. Drink about 64 ounces of water a day. But if you work out hard, drink more than that. If the weather is dry and hot, or if you are sweating profusely, drink liberally. Water by itself won't sculpt your body, but it keeps your metabolism revved.

YOUR PERSONAL TRAINER

Limit your soft drink consumption and drink water instead. The average can of your favorite soft drink contains about 10 teaspoons of sugar. Replace sugared drinks immediately and within a couple weeks you will see changes in your body just from doing that.

It's almost impossible to drink too much water. Drink enough water so that your urine is clear, and that you feel a need to relieve yourself every two hours. Water helps to speed up the cellulite-burning process and aid your metabolism. Water is your first choice of liquid fuel, but if you must substitute, drink flavored water.

Your Daily Diet

You should consider adjusting your nutritional intake, time, frequency, and so on according to your schedule and activities. Figure out the foods that work for you. You may prefer to eat most of your starchy carbs through the day and cut back on them in the evening. Eat breakfast like a king, lunch like a queen, and dinner like a pauper.

Eating breakfast is an important part of a healthy diet. After fasting all night, your muscles need energy. Eating breakfast not only increases your energy, but you will make better food choices for the rest of the day. A good breakfast is oatmeal or a low-sugar cold cereal, nonfat milk, and a banana or raisins.

Eat a turkey or lean roast beef sandwich for lunch, replacing the mayonnaise for mustard or horseradish. Between lunch and dinner try some sliced fruit with cottage cheese. Dinner can be fish, rice, salad with a drizzle of healthy dressing, and your favorite fruit.

Eat before you are hungry, drink before you are thirsty. Never let yourself go more than a couple hours without sustenance. If you don't eat now, you may eat too much later.

IN OTHER WORDS

Under-eating leads to cheating. Don't skip meals. Craving sweets may mean that you are not eating enough throughout the day.

Regular snacks between meals assure that your system won't cannibalize your hard-earned toned body. A perfect snack is a combination of carbs and protein. Your favorite fruit and cottage cheese or peanut butter and a banana are good choices.

Spend a few minutes each evening planning the next day's meals and snacks. Examine your schedule. Figure out when you get hungry and have appropriate snacks available. Carry a cooler in your car filled with plastic containers of your favorite foods. Pack peanut butter on whole-wheat bread, yogurt, and a banana; pita bread with hummus, baby carrots, and a green pepper. Keep your desk drawer stocked with nuts, pretzels, dried fruit, and oatmeal.

> **IN OTHER WORDS**
>
> Simple carbs that have a high glycemic index travel from your stomach to your bloodstream to your muscles, liver, or fat stores very quickly.

Don't be afraid to special-order at restaurants. Ask that your foods be poached, grilled, steamed, or baked. Request that the chef not add extra oil, cream, or butter in your dishes. Some "special sauces" are very high in calories. Remember to order dressing on the side, so *you* control how much you will eat.

It is better to be disciplined about your eating than fanatical. Choose round steak instead of hamburger; pork loin instead of bacon; baked potatoes, rice, and beans instead of French fries, fried rice, and refried beans.

What if you need to eat 2,000 calories a day to maintain your metabolism? It's 10:00 p.m. and so far you have only eaten 1,500 calories. Should you go to bed hungry, or eat 500 more calories?

The answer is: Don't go to bed hungry. Have a reasonable, healthy 500-calorie mini-meal to ensure that your muscles stay nourished.

Eat to Feed Your Muscles

What you learned in health class and from your mother is still true: *a balanced diet of fruits and veggies is good for you.* Add a portion of lean protein with a tablespoon of your favorite healthy essential fat and you're on your way to that sculpted body you deserve. Think of a round plate cut in thirds. One third is a lean protein, one third is a fruit, and one third is a vegetable.

Three things happen to the calories you eat. Either they are burned up by your metabolism or activity, stored in your muscle, or stored as fat. Try eating small meals throughout the day instead of a couple large ones. Your fat cells are a lot less likely to fill up if you eat mini-meals because your body has immediate energy to draw from. If you eat large quantities of food in a single sitting, your body stores what it doesn't need at the moment. And yes, your body will store this extra energy as fat. A few hours later, you will be hungry again, even though your fat stores are full.

Use the eating-frequency plan that works best for you and your particular lifestyle. A midmorning mini-meal helps stabilize blood sugar so you won't be ravenous at lunch, but if you eat a huge breakfast of eggs, whole-wheat toast, and oatmeal, you may not need a snack between breakfast and lunch.

GET IT RIGHT

Eat until you're full or you'll be tempted to eat something that isn't so good for you. If your body hasn't received enough nutrients, it'll let you know through hunger pangs, tiredness, and so on.

When you eat food your body must work hard to digest it. When your body works hard it uses up calories. Eating breakfast-snack-lunch-snack-dinner keeps your metabolism revved all day long. You are constantly feeding your muscle so you don't have to worry about muscle being used for energy.

After eating correctly becomes a habit, you will look forward to feeding your muscles quality food every few hours. Eat right most of the time and you are on the program. You will have bad eating days and that's okay. Bad days are part of the eating program. It's about getting back on track again and again that makes your eating program a success.

Eat to Fuel Your Workouts

Fueling your workout is a major part of seeing great definition in your body. What you eat today and tomorrow will benefit your workouts the next day and the day after that.

Your muscles are 70 percent water. Before you begin your training, drink 2 cups of water. To keep your muscles full and tight, begin drinking 6 ounces of water every 20 minutes throughout your workout.

Balancing your meals energizes your workouts. You may burn between 300 and 500 calories per training session. Therefore, be sure you are eating enough to maintain your hard-earned muscle. Eat four carbs to one protein as soon after your workout as you can to speed nutrients to your depleted muscles.

Eat real food! You don't need to buy expensive supplements; they don't make up for poor eating habits. Unlike tablet supplements, fruits and vegetables offer far more than just vitamins. They also contain fiber and other compounds that are essential to a healthy body. Feed your muscles and starve your fat.

GET IT RIGHT

Eat for the right reasons. Most people eat for reasons other than hunger. For one month, develop the mentality that you're going to eat to fuel your workouts. After a month, you can do whatever you like. You'll be amazed at the difference this makes in how you approach eating, because you won't want to lose the great results you achieved in that one month.

After your workout, grab a sports drink or glass of juice to energize worn-out muscles. Include a little protein in your after-workout snack, too, because working out tears down muscle tissue, and protein rebuilds muscle. Pair a tuna on whole-wheat sandwich with a glass of juice or sports drink.

Your depleted muscles need energy to return to normal function. Consuming protein and carbs after a workout will also aid in repairing and rebuilding muscle, and replenish the glycogen stores you need. Look for a sports drink with between 10 and 20 grams of carbohydrates per 8-ounce serving. Your next workout will feel easier if you refuel your muscle as soon as you have completed that last set of squats.

The quantity of food you eat before and after your workout depends on your metabolism and your activity. The harder the activity, the more calories you need. If you want to be scientific, eat at least 10 times your body weight in calories to maintain your hard-earned muscle. If you weigh 150 pounds, eat at least 1,500 calories throughout the day. Try having a snack before your workout and see if that helps you move a little farther or get a few extra reps.

The more you work out and the harder each workout is, the more food you need. If you walk a mile, that burns about 100 calories. If you take an indoor cycling class, count on burning at least 450 calories. There are all kinds of formulas to try and determine how many calories you should eat, depending on your metabolism.

If you are moderately active—for example, you walk 30 minutes four days a week and lift weights twice a week—then multiply your body weight by 13. The number you come up with equals the minimum number of calories you should eat each day just to support your metabolism.

Eat to Starve Your Fat Cells

If you don't eat enough, your metabolism slows and your body holds on to your fat stores. If you eat too much, you add extra insulation around your brand-new muscles.

If you deprive yourself of a certain type of food, you will want it more. Rather than eat all of the health food in your house and then succumb to the "forbidden" item, you could go ahead and satisfy your craving immediately. On the other hand, if you know that a "trigger food" will set off a binge, then don't start at all. The best way to eliminate trigger foods is to not have them in your home.

To inspire you to stay with your healthy eating program, pinch the fat on the back of your upper arm, on the side of your waist, or on your inner thigh. Grab an inch of fat between your thumb and index finger and then decide if you really need to eat. Or decide if the food you are about to eat will fuel your muscle or add to your fat stores.

YOUR PERSONAL TRAINER

A pocket spiral notebook will help you determine if you are eating right or cheating too much.

Eating perfectly all of the time is no fun, and nobody eats right 100 percent of the time. "Keep progressing, not perfecting" is the mantra of healthy eating. It has nothing to do with willpower; it just requires some thought and planning. Plan your meals in advance and have the discipline to eat every few hours.

You'll know when you lose that extra fat. You'll feel better. Don't worry about what the scale says. Instead, focus on how your clothes fit. You won't be afraid to wear sleeveless shirts, shorts, or a bathing suit. When your clothes fit looser and your energy level increases, you are on the program for life.

The Least You Need to Know

- Eat nutrient-dense carbs instead of calorically dense carbs.
- Keep a food journal to track your eating habits and make improvements.
- Expect not to eat perfectly all the time, but always strive to get right back to healthy eating after a slip up.
- Eating several small meals and drinking lots of water are essential to maintaining a healthy diet.

Putting It All Together

In This Chapter

- Adding more activity to your day
- Learning how to split up your workouts
- Starting your healthy eating program

If getting a toned and defined body meant spending a couple hours a day working out, more people would have a sculpted body. It's not just about working out.

To get the body you want, put it all together: eat right, stay active, and do isolation exercises in the areas you want to strengthen and tone. You will see results fast if you combine all three aspects of this total body program.

And it's not that hard. The hardest part of the workout is turning off that computer. Finding the time to work out is an art. A few minutes of exercise, several times a day, boosts energy, decreases stress, builds confidence, and helps you sleep better. So if you can sneak five minutes several times a day, you will get more of your computer work done in a shorter period.

Increase Your Activity

Just move. After you start moving it becomes a habit. Soon it will feel excruciating to sit for long periods. Your body loves to move, so let it!

No exercise gizmo is better than simply moving your body against gravity. Move at different angles and intensities to burn more calories.

Listen to your body. Talk with your physician about any tweaks or creaks that last more than a week. Stay below the symptoms of any discomfort or pain.

Add Twenty Minutes a Day

If you can work your way up to moving an extra 20 minutes each day, you are *guaranteed* to make progress. You don't have to move fast, just move.

Take the stairs instead of the elevator and park in the space furthest from your office. Make your life one mini-workout after another instead of finding ways to sit.

Don't work up a sweat, but move. If you have to sit, and no one is watching, punch an imaginary boxing speed bag by rolling your hands around each other above your head.

Keep track of how many extra minutes you move each day. If you haven't reached 20 extra minutes by dinnertime, go for a quick walk.

BET YOU DIDN'T KNOW

A muscle cell weighs more than a fat cell, but a fat cell is almost five times larger than a muscle cell.

You may decide to use a pedometer that attaches to your belt like a pager. It keeps track of how many steps you take each day. Aim for about 10,000 steps a day.

Although you have probably heard these suggestions before, they really work. Shedding fat is a cumulative effort.

Train yourself to move instead of being still. Be creative about adding movement into your day. When your exercise is a pleasure, developing your abs will be easy.

Add Five Minutes a Week

Twenty minutes of extra activity each day is your first step toward seeing better definition in your body. Your next step is to add five minutes of movement each week. In just eight weeks, you will be moving an hour a day beyond what you were doing before. By then you will have the sculpted body you've been hoping for.

> **IN OTHER WORDS**
>
> Crossing your anaerobic threshold or lactate threshold means that you are no longer training at a steady state. You have crossed over the line and are huffing and puffing and burning.

If your boss allows you to sit on an exercise ball instead of a chair, you burn extra calories just keeping your balance. Instead of using email, walk a few steps to your colleague's office and deliver the message in person.

The more you move, the higher your energy level. With increased energy, you move more. It's a cycle of progress that trims your body in no time.

Move Your Body

You burn similar calories whether you walk a mile or jog a mile, so why not take it easy? Some people think that there is something magic about running and losing weight. Walking briskly burns even more calories than a slow jog.

If you want to maintain your upper-body muscles, abs, and lower-body muscles, walk instead of run. Pounding the pavement actually breaks down your hard-earned muscle. You probably don't want the body of a marathon runner, so don't train like one. Too much aerobic activity breaks down muscle tissue, and you don't want that.

Stick with nonimpact activities such as stair climbing, elliptical machines, cross-country skiing, and cycling. Do the minimum amount of cardio—30 to 45 minutes, three or four days a week. When you do too much cardio, your body uses your muscle tissue for energy. So take it down a notch.

To discover if you are doing too much cardio or working out too hard, take notice of your strength levels. If you remain strong and your upper-, mid-, and lower-body muscles are sculpted and toned, you are doing fine.

IN OTHER WORDS

Train according to your *perceived exertion*. Perceived exertion is a measure of how hard you are training based on how you feel.

Accessorize

Dress for success in your workouts. Comfortable, supportive, breathable clothes are important to melting fat and toning your body. The most important part of your exercise wardrobe is your shoes. If your feet don't feel good, you'll find a reason to stop moving. Take a look at your shoes before you begin. Don't wear your old tennis shoes. Purchase a shoe that supports the type of activity you choose. Because you want to avoid impact activities, get a good, supportive walking shoe for the trails or treadmills. A walking shoe is specially designed with added flexibility in the ball of the foot to "toe-off" on each step.

A cross-training shoe will be fine for pedaling, stepping, or gliding. When you find a pair you like, buy an identical pair for the office. Then over your lunch break, you can walk up the stairs of your office building and take the elevator down for a nonimpact workout.

Get in the Mood

Training your body in the weight room requires concentration. If you zone out during your weight workouts, you won't achieve the body of your dreams. But your mental state for easy activity is a different story. Movement is a mood improver, and even just walking will lift your spirits. If you don't enjoy being alone with your thoughts, take headphones on your walk. Get pumped up with your favorite tunes. But don't let the music inspire you to a level of activity that breaks down your precious muscle tissue.

Working Out in Intervals

After your toning workout, your metabolism stays revved for several minutes. The same is true after you complete your cardio workout.

IN OTHER WORDS

Excess postexercise oxygen consumption (EPOC) is the afterburn—the extra amount of calories your body continues to burn after you have completed your workout.

Interval training is a way to burn calories fast. And if you burn a lot of calories, you lose a lot of fat. On all of these interval activity programs, stay below the level of huffing and puffing and burning. Warm up for five minutes before you begin and cool down for five minutes at the completion of your workout.

If you reside near a track, try this interval recipe. After your warm-up, walk the length of the track briskly at 70 percent of your maximum effort. Walk slowly around the curve. Do this for 5 cycles. Be sure to cool down with some slow walking and easy stretching when you have completed your workout.

Here are a couple other programs to change up your workouts and keep you progressing. Begin with easy movement, then gradually step it up. Moving fast simply means moving at a pace that is challenging but doable.

Program 1: Begin with a 5-minute warm-up of easy movement and always finish with a 5-minute cool-down. During Week One, move for 25 minutes doing a 3-minute fast interval and a 1-minute slow interval. During Week Two, move for 30 minutes doing a 4-minute fast interval and a 1-minute slow interval.

Program 2: Recreational intervals are fun. You speed up and slow down depending on how you feel. If you're ready to pick up the pace, go for it. If you are breathless, slow down. Although recreational intervals are not structured, the benefits are the same as regular intervals.

Interval training is not magic. Don't try intervals every time you move. In fact, it's better to train according to how you feel. If you love doing intervals, have at it. If not, stay with your favorite easy activity. Moving slowly is a lot better than not moving at all.

GET IT RIGHT

Don't get caught up with thinking you must have a sensational workout every time you hit the pavement. Everyone has off days.

Isolation Training

You can perform your isolation training at home, in your office, or in the gym. Train your muscles no more than twice a week, but with at least 48 hours rest in between workouts. Your exercises should take no longer than a few minutes.

How hard you train your muscles is more important than how long. Go for the burn occasionally, but if your muscles feel uncomfortable for a couple days afterward, you went too far.

YOUR PERSONAL TRAINER

Choose the routine that works for you. Push one day, pull the next. Or try chest, back, and shoulders one day and arms the next day. When you stop making progress, it's time to change your program.

What Works for You

If you prefer to minimize your workout time, just train each area twice a week. But if you love to train, you can do a split routine. A split routine means that you will train a couple times a day on the same area.

If you enjoy working out daily, you can train several days a week using a split routine. Perform 3 sets of 10 repetitions of each exercise with perfect form. Your first set is a warm-up and your second and third sets are working sets.

Remember to mix and match. Your muscles need to be challenged from different angles and intensities for them to grow. Use perfect form to maximize your progress and minimize soreness.

YOUR PERSONAL TRAINER

If you are extremely short on time at home or in the gym, do supersets. This routine keeps your heart rate up so that your muscles get toned and streamlined simultaneously. Focusing on one area of the body, perform a set of 10 reps of one exercise, then without rest do another set of 10 of a different exercise. Do 3 sets, take a one-minute break, and then repeat with two other exercises in the same body area.

Add Two Reps a Week

When you first begin training, your body responds to almost any exercise you do, especially women. When they begin training, they improve at least as fast as men.

But if you don't challenge your muscles, they stay the same. That is why you should add weight when you can complete 10 repetitions with perfect form. Look for visible results in a few weeks.

Add One Exercise a Month

Just as you get bored doing the same exercises, your muscles do, too. When you don't add anything new to your muscle-isolation programs, don't expect to see improvement. Adding one new exercise each month will ignite your progress.

GET IT RIGHT

Do not stretch your working muscles vigorously between sets. Wait to stretch until after the workout. Instead, use that time to mentally prepare for your next set.

Your Healthy Eating Program

Anybody can go on an exercise program, but changing your eating habits is the key to seeing your new body emerge.

Miracle diets return every seven years with different names. The Atkins low-carb diet is similar to Dr. Stillman's diet in the 1960s, which required you to eat meat, cheese, and eggs.

Liquid diets have come and gone and so have the single-food (grapefruit, cabbage), all-you-can-eat plans.

GET IT RIGHT

Subtract 250 calories more each day from your diet and in a week you will lose half a pound. It doesn't sound like much, but by using another 250 calories in exercise, you can lose about 2 pounds of flab in a week.

There is no doubt that you can lose weight on diets that limit you to a few food groups, but you cannot keep the weight off. So get back to the basics and do it right. Make eating right part of your lifestyle instead of "going on a diet."

Eating After Your Workout

Eat half a gram of carbohydrate per pound of body weight within three hours of your workout. If you weigh 150 pounds, you should eat a quick 75 grams of carbohydrate (1 banana) and 19 grams of protein (2 cups of nonfat milk). Eat to fuel your muscles. After you work out, you should eat a 4:1 ratio of carbs to protein as soon as possible to replenish glycogen stores and rebuild muscle. Not only will you feel better, you will have more energy and your arms will thank you.

Following is a partial list of foods for your eating program. This is just a quick sample; what you choose really depends on your taste.

GET IT RIGHT

Eat a substantial breakfast and it will power your workout and energize your day.

Mix and match a lean protein, complex carbohydrate, and fruit for each meal and snack throughout the day.

Sample Foods on the Eating Program

Lean Protein	Complex Carbs	Fruit
Turkey	Cruciferous veggies	Strawberries
Pork loin	Cereals	Blueberries
Dairy	Whole grains	Raspberries
Fish	Corn family	Apricots
Venison	Salad family	Bananas
Buffalo	Lentils	Pineapple

Lots of Water

Water is the ultimate nutrient. Approximately 70 percent of the body is water. Water does not provide energy, but it is involved in just about every process in the human body. Eight glasses of water a day are enough for sedentary couch potatoes, but not for you.

Drink about 1 milliliter of water per calorie that you burn. That means if you burn 2,000 calories working out, you need to drink an additional 2 liters of water.

Essential, Omega-3 Fats

Omega-3 fats from fish and unsaturated fat from oils are part of a body-toning diet.

Eat dietary fat as 15 to 20 percent of your total calories. For men, that is about 60 grams of fat on a 2,500-calorie diet. Women should take in about 40 grams of fat on a 2,000-calorie diet. Your activity level helps determine the amount of calories and fat to consume.

It Works

This eating program is your dream come true. You eat before you are hungry and you drink a lot of water throughout the day. Never let yourself go more than a few hours without food. Choose foods that you love. There are no forbidden foods; you eat what you like in moderation. Prepare your foods in advance so that you know what you are going to eat tomorrow.

Feed your workouts with a combination of lean protein, starchy carbohydrates, and fibrous vegetables. When in doubt, always choose whole foods and natural fruits and vegetables instead of man-made, processed, and hydrogenated products. Take a day off from the eating program once a week—that is part of the program. If you give yourself permission to have a treat now and then, you're less likely to binge and fall off the wagon. You'll just get back on the program for your next meal.

The Least You Need to Know

- Increase the amount of time you are active by 20 minutes a day.
- Add more reps and exercises to your regimen each month to continue your progress.
- Steer clear of fad diets and consistently stick with whole, all-natural foods.

Upper Body

This part provides exercises that will cut and define the muscles in your chest, back, shoulders, and arms. You will learn upper-body workouts you can do at the gym, at home, even at the office, as well as stretches to keep you flexible and feeling good.

Upper Body Made Simple

In This Chapter

- The major muscles in the upper body
- The upper body results men and women seek
- The best way to remember your back
- The path to broader shoulders is not a dream

Ever notice someone with a great upper body walking through the mall? Your eyes are drawn to well-defined arms, a broad chest, and a tapered, V-shaped back.

Changing the shape of your upper body isn't brain surgery, and you can have that sculpted upper body, too. Evaluate your upper body in a mirror. Decide if you want to shape and slenderize your arms and shoulders, lift up that chest, and/or firm your back. Be specific about the changes you would like to make according to the anatomy presented in this chapter.

Males usually want to increase the size and density of their upper-body muscles. It's hard to find a man who doesn't want a big chest and strong arms. Women prefer an athletic, shapely, firm, and feminine body. A well-proportioned, sleek, and defined upper body is ideal.

Good genes may provide you with a great figure, but you have to earn defined muscles. The purpose of this chapter is to help you design the ideal shape for your upper body. Sure, genetics play a role, but you can improve each of your upper-body muscle groups, increase the separation between each muscle, and enhance the detail of your entire upper body.

GET IT RIGHT

There are three basic body types: endomorph, a heavy, rounded appearance; ectomorph, very thin; and mesomorph, V-shaped and muscular. Although you cannot change the shape of your muscles, you can sculpt them to create the best-shaped upper body your genetic potential will allow.

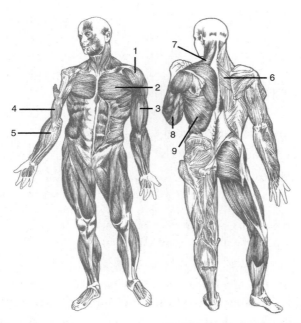

1. Deltoid (shoulder)
2. Pectoralis major (chest)
3. Biceps brachii (front upper arm)
4. Brachialis (side upper arm)
5. Brachioradialis (upper arm and forearm)

6. Rhomboids (middle back)
7. Trapezius (upper shoulder)
8. Triceps brachii (back upper arm)
9. Latissimus dorsi (upper back)

The muscle groups in your upper body.

Arms

The upper arms consist of two muscle groups, the biceps and the triceps. The biceps run along the front of the upper arms and are responsible for bending the elbow. The triceps run along the back of the arm.

Biceps

When it comes to arm training, men have an obsession with the biceps. To be able to fold up your sleeves and display peaked, rock hard, striated upper arms, is one of the greatest sensations of the male ego. Men want big biceps because they are visible in the mirror and attract the attention of others—not just from the opposite sex, but also among their peers.

Make a muscle by bending your elbow and bringing your fist toward your shoulder. The biceps consist of an inner and outer head on the top side of your upper arm. The *biceps brachii* is your beach muscle. Although some people can make this muscle peak at the top when they flex it, genetics plays a huge role in the actual shape of the muscle.

The *brachialis muscle* is underneath your biceps and adds fullness to your arm. You can see this muscle better from a side view.

YOUR PERSONAL TRAINER

Spend more time focusing your training on your major muscle groups (chest, back, and shoulders) instead of worrying about your arms. When you train your large muscle groups, your arms are working, too.

Triceps

Women are concerned less about the size of their biceps and more about firmness and definition. The focal point of female upper-arm training is the triceps in the back of the arm.

Well-defined triceps are very attractive. A toned set of triceps creates an image of youth, vitality, and sexiness. Everyone wants to bare his or her arms and be buffed and tank top–ready. Well-toned triceps are a perfect warm-weather accessory. With a little effort, sculpted triceps are within your reach.

The triceps run along the back of the upper arm. Their purpose is to extend the elbow to straighten the arm. Your triceps muscles are almost double the size of your biceps.

The triceps are two thirds of the muscle mass of your upper arms. Because your triceps has three heads and your biceps only two, your biceps will never catch up to your triceps; nor should they.

Extend your elbows to the front with your palms facing down. Find a mirror and look at the back of your upper arms. Your defined triceps are shaped like miniature horseshoes.

Back

One of the first mistakes people make when training the upper body is to train the muscles they can see—chest and arms. Your chest and arms are small muscle groups compared to your back. They don't have as much potential for adding a visual change to your body.

The back muscles are neglected because you don't see them every day, but your back is important in creating an overall symmetrical physique that is pleasing to the eye. Women want a toned back because it helps them stand taller and stop that nagging bra-strap bulge. A V-back silhouette gives the appearance of a narrow waist and smaller hips, as well as creating the illusion that your arms are more developed.

Feel the widest part of your back just behind your armpit. Those are your *latissimus dorsi* muscles, or lats. The lats are the largest back muscles, and the ones that give most of the "V-taper" to your upper body. Your lats run the entire length of your back from your shoulders to your hips. Well-toned lats add shape and width to your upper body. A lat spread that fans out resembles a cobra's head. If you develop your lats, your friends will notice immediately.

Another important set of back muscles is the *rhomboids*. These are small rectangular muscles at the center of your back just beneath your shoulders. They are named after the geometric parallelogram with no right angles and adjacent sides of unequal length. They have two parts, a major and minor, and are located on both sides of the upper part of your spine.

If you work at a desk all day, you probably round your back. Pull your shoulders back and down. Your rhomboids are the muscles that did most of the work. Sloppy posture is unattractive, so a poised, confident look is important. Your rhomboids are one of the major muscle groups responsible for maintaining perfect upper-body posture. Flex your rhomboids and your shoulders stay back and your chest naturally extends outward. Your rhomboids counteract the tendency to hunch your shoulders. You feel better and look better with strong, toned rhomboids.

Shoulders

Whether you're fat or thin, dressed for work or for the beach, wide shoulders give a powerful impression. Broad shoulders are the most visible part of your "X-frame." Your shoulders are the top of the "V" created by your sleek back. Great-looking shoulders hide possible flaws in your waist and the rest of your upper body. Broad shoulders combined with a V-back create the illusion of a smaller waist, even if your waist size doesn't change.

To see just how much of a difference this makes, take a pair of socks and stuff them inside your shirt on each side of your shoulders. Then look in the mirror. Even a small increase in width completely transforms your appearance.

IN OTHER WORDS

You have four rotator cuff muscles that attach your shoulder to your upper arm bone. They are your supra-spinatus, infraspinatus, teres minor, and subscapularis.

Shapely shoulders can be yours with a little effort. Cup your right hand on your left shoulder. Raise your left hand toward the ceiling and you can feel your shoulder muscles flex. Any pressing movement over your head involves your shoulders.

Your shoulder muscles, or *deltoids*, have three parts: medial, anterior, and posterior. Feel your medial deltoids by raising your arms from your sides as if you were doing slow-motion jumping jacks. This is the muscle that widens your X-frame, and, if you train hard enough, will make the sides of your shoulders the size of softballs.

Flex the front of your shoulder (anterior deltoid) by raising your arm to the front. The anterior deltoid muscles are visible just to the outside of your chest muscles. When these muscles are defined, it's hard to take your eyes off of them.

Don't forget to train the back of your shoulder (posterior deltoid). The posterior deltoids look awesome when they are cut and defined. They are located further back on your shoulder, just above your shoulder blade. These muscles make an impression when someone sees you from behind.

Traps

It is important for you to identify each set of shoulder muscles so you can increase them, tone them, or leave them alone. You have a nice-sized chest, well-defined delts, and your lats are so wide your elbows don't touch your sides anymore. But the mirror tells you that something is missing. Your head and neck don't seem to have a solid base of support.

This is where your *trapezius* (traps) comes in. Your traps are a set of muscles that are often overlooked, because they're not in your immediate vision. You don't recognize them as a separate muscle because you use them when you train almost every other upper-body part.

Your traps are thick, triangular muscles that run from your neck across the top of the shoulder, and down along your backbone to the middle of your back. These kite-shaped muscles are the largest muscle group in your upper shoulder. A toned set of traps adds shape to your shoulders and upper back.

Use your traps to shrug your shoulders. Your traps also work with your deltoids to raise your hand. If your traps become too large you might begin to resemble a cartoon character.

BET YOU DIDN'T KNOW

If a muscle becomes too large, stop training it. If a muscle is not used, it atrophies. Use it or lose it.

Chest

A wimpy chest detracts from an impressive upper body. An undefined chest makes you look older than your years. A sculpted chest appears attractive even if your lower body carries more fat than it should.

A broad chest is perhaps the most widely sought muscle group of the human physique. It is rare to find a gym-goer, particularly a male, who isn't looking to put another inch or two on the chest. It is the body part that even skinny guys on the beach try to develop.

Place your right hand on your left chest muscle. Push your desk with your left hand. Feel the chest muscles stimulated by the pushing movement. Now place your right hand on your left chest muscle. This time, move your left arm horizontally, back and forth. Your chest muscles flex when you bring your arm toward the middle of your body.

Ideal chest development is not a hanging, bulbous mass, but muscles that are fully defined from top to bottom. The chest muscles run all the way from your collarbone to just below your nipple.

For guys with low body fat, the chest muscles cut a sharp, flaring line clearly delineating the outer and lower chest border. The chest muscles are fan-shaped, and the outer and lower fibers are one and the same muscle.

Your chest muscles are referred to as pectoral muscles. The *pectoralis major* can be felt under the breast when the muscle is flexed. The *pectoralis minor* is near your collarbone on the upper chest.

The pectoralis major is larger and attaches to the sternum. The pectoralis minor connects to the collarbone. Both pectoralis muscles are surrounded by the collarbone, sternum, and ribcage, and are attached to the upper-arm bone.

The Least You Need to Know

- The upper body is comprised of arms, chest, back, shoulders, and traps.
- Don't neglect training your back just because you can't see it.
- Broad shoulders are desirable because they make the waist look smaller.
- A well-defined chest gives a youthful appearance.

Upper Body at Home

In This Chapter

- The convenience of upper-body workouts at home
- The most effective push-ups and dips
- The way to target your chest and back
- The shoulder workout

There's no place like home for training convenience. You don't have to drive any-where, the weather is never a problem, and you don't have to worry about parking. Best of all, you can exercise in your pajamas and no one will care. At home, you don't have to talk to anyone. If you feel uncomfortable around hard bodies, you won't have to see them, either. And you may not enjoy working out around people of the oppo-site sex. You don't have to wait for machines or hear the endless clanging of weights, and you don't have to wipe sweat off machines. At home there are fewer distractions than in the gym. Most importantly, you won't have a monthly gym payment.

No gym equipment is necessary to develop firm arms, a tapered back, and a well-defined chest. On all tone-at-home upper-body exercises, keep your back straight, stomach in, neck relaxed, and head up. Perform each exercise three seconds up and three seconds down through a full range of motion. Perform 10 repetitions of each exercise exhaling on the exertion phase of each rep. Focus on the muscles you are training and relax the others. If an exercise is too difficult, choose another one.

Modified Push-Ups

Modified Push-Ups are the best exercise for your upper body. You firm your chest, back, arms, and shoulders. The rest of your body has to support your movement, too.

Keep your back straight and knees slightly bent so that a straight line can be drawn from the back of your head to the back of your heels. At first, don't concern yourself with how far you descend. The up position is a workout in itself. As you get stronger, go down further until eventually your elbows bend at 90 degrees.

Do not rest in the up or the down position. Do not fully extend your elbows in the up position. Your elbows should always remain soft (slightly bent). Move slowly through each repetition so that if you stop at any point during the rep, you maintain perfect form.

Be careful that your back doesn't sag as you fatigue. Lead with your chest and resist the temptation to drop your head. Your head should always stay in line with your spine. Begin doing modified push-ups on the wall. When you can do 10 repetitions with perfect form, do them from the floor on your knees. When you can do 10 reps with perfect form, try them from your feet. You can also use a stability ball to make the exercise easier or more difficult.

1. Your hands are shoulder-width apart on the wall or on the floor. If you are on the floor, you may begin on your knees or on your feet.

2. Lower your chest a few inches by bending your elbows 90 degrees.

3. Return to your starting position by extending your elbows.

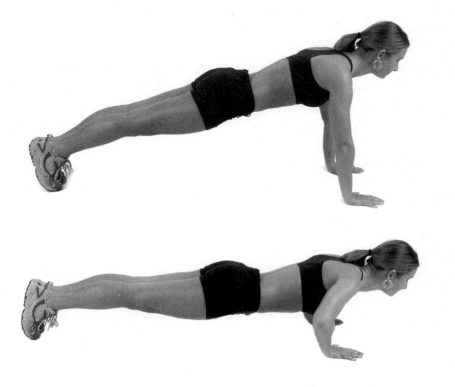

IN OTHER WORDS

Your pectoralis major and pectoralis minor muscles are the muscles of your chest. They may be toned and tightened from several different angles.

Close Grip Push-Ups

Close Grip Push-Ups zone in on the backs of your arms and the fronts of your shoulders. This is one of the best exercises for the backs of your arms.

The back of your body should be a perfectly slanted ramp from the top of your head to the back of your heel. Don't allow your head to drop or move to either side. Your head should always stay in line with your spine.

Lead with your chest on each repetition. Keep your upper arms near your sides. Do not allow your elbows to flare out or lock in the up position. If your wrists or elbows hurt when you perform this exercise, spread your hands out until you are pain-free. Do not rest in the up or the down position. Keep your elbows in close to your body and your back straight throughout the duration of the exercise.

BET YOU DIDN'T KNOW

Any movement where you flex your elbows in a pulling motion tones the fronts of your arms. Any movement that extends your elbows tones the backs of your arms.

1. Your hands are together creating a diamond shape with your fingers on the wall or on the floor. If you are on the floor, you may begin on your knees or on your feet.

2. Lower your chest a few inches by bending your elbows to a 90-degree angle, keeping the elbows close to the body.

3. Return to your starting position by extending your elbows.

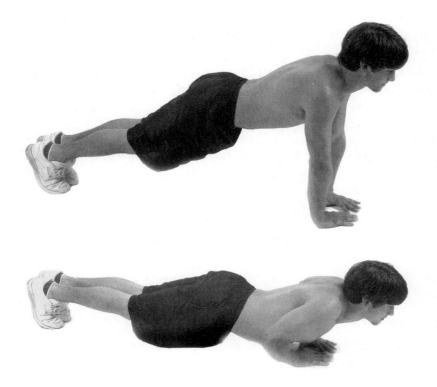

Chair Dips

Dips tighten the backs of your arms, chest, and shoulders. Don't round your back or bend your elbows too much. Keep your back straight, elbows in, shoulders down, and chest out.

GET IT RIGHT

To preserve your shoulder joints, do all exercises in front of the neck instead of behind the neck. For all exercises there is a risk versus benefit. There is no reason to do any exercise pressing from behind the neck because of possible rotator cuff damage and cervical spine injury. And for triceps, the load puts too much stress on a hyper-flexed elbow. There is no need to flex the elbow beyond 90 degrees to train the triceps. A great rule of thumb is that you should always be able to see your hands during any exercise.

Begin each exercise by drawing your navel into your spine. At first, bend your arms only slightly for each rep. As you get stronger, bend your arms further until you max out at 90 degrees. Never bend your elbows further than 90 degrees. In the up position, keep your elbows soft.

If this exercise is too difficult, allow your legs to boost you back into the up position on each rep. An advanced form of this exercise would be to place a weight in your lap when you perform your repetitions.

1. Sit on the edge of a chair with your hands behind you and your palms facing downward.

2. Keep your hands shoulder-width apart and extend your legs out to the front.

3. Brace yourself with your hands as you lower yourself a few inches by bending your elbows.

4. Return to your original position by extending your elbows.

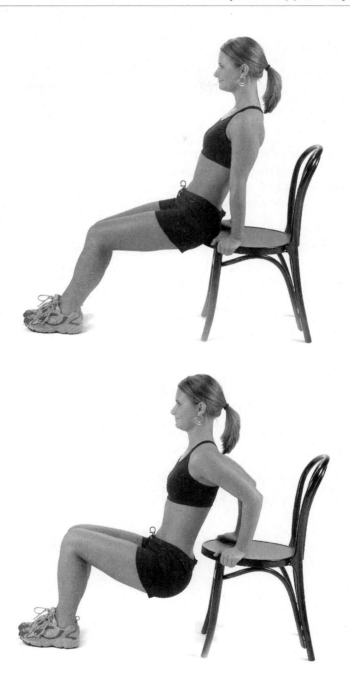

Chest Fly on Floor

The Chest Fly on Floor shapes up your chest. Begin each exercise by drawing your navel into your spine. Flex your chest muscles as you move through your range of motion. Imagine flexing your chest muscles together so that a nickel wouldn't fall out from between them.

Concentrate on flexing your chest on both the upward and the downward motion to get maximum results. Keep your elbows bent at all times and be sure that both arms move together. Shoulders should stay down and your head should rest on the floor. When you can perform 10 repetitions with perfect form, add more weight.

YOUR PERSONAL TRAINER

If you have a twinge of discomfort as you move through any exercise, find a different range of motion to prevent pain and possible injury.

1. Lie on your back with your arms out to the side with your elbows slightly bent. Hold a light can in each hand.

2. Bring your arms together toward the middle of your chest as if you were hugging a tree—not too straight or bent, just a slight curve at the elbow.

3. Return to your original position, bringing your arms in the same path that you did when you brought them together.

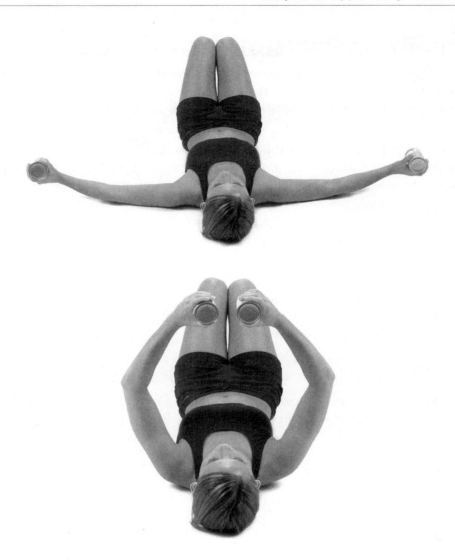

Single Arm Rowing with Chair

The Single Arm Rowing with Chair gives your back that hourglass shape. Begin in a position of stability. Draw your navel into your spine. Keep your upper body square to the floor for the duration of the exercise. Resist the temptation to twist your upper body.

The first movement you make should be your shoulder blade moving toward the ceiling. It is particularly important on this exercise not to jerk the weight up. Be sure to keep your back tabletop flat and don't bring your elbow up too high.

GET IT RIGHT

Be careful not to fully extend your elbows or knees on any exercise, as that takes the resistance off your muscles and puts pressure on your joints.

1. Stand next to a chair and bend from your hips with your left hand supporting your body on the chair and your right arm extended by your side. Keep your back straight during the entire exercise. Hold on to a can with your right hand.

2. Pull the can up to your side by lifting your elbow toward the ceiling.

3. Return to the starting position moving your arm along the same path.

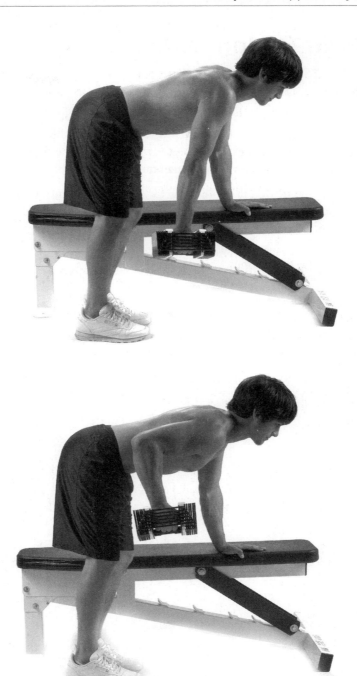

Lateral Arm Raise

The Lateral Arm Raise builds the sides of your shoulders. You may never have to wear shoulder pads again. Perform this exercise seated or standing.

Begin by drawing your navel into your spine. Keep your back straight and move slowly so that you are not throwing the weights. You should be able to stop at any point during the lift and maintain perfect form. Keep your elbows slightly bent throughout the movement and bring your hands no higher than shoulder level.

If this exercise is too difficult, lighten the weight or bend your elbows 90 degrees. To make this exercise more challenging, extend your elbows until they are just slightly bent. For further isolation, you may perform all of your repetitions with one arm and then repeat with your other arm.

1. Begin by sitting with your feet shoulder-width apart and your arms held to your sides with your elbows slightly bent.

2. Keep your elbows bent as you raise both arms up from your sides until they are parallel to the floor.

3. Return to your original position, keeping your arms moving in the same path.

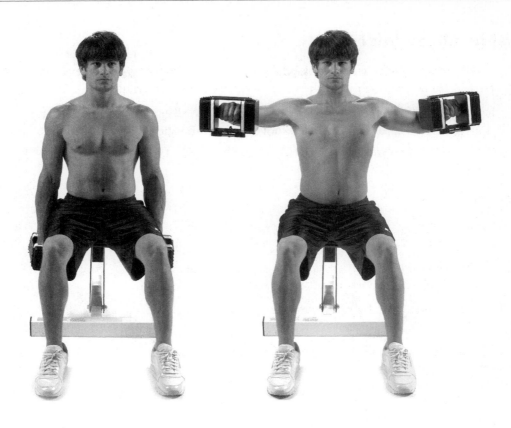

The Least You Need to Know

- Weights, a chair, and/or a bench are all you need to tone your upper body at home.
- A straight back is essential for effective push-ups.
- Always use slow, controlled movements with weights.
- Add more weight when you can perform a set of reps in perfect form.

Upper Body at the Office

In This Chapter

- Working out at work
- Toning with desk push-ups and dips
- Working the shoulders and back from your chair
- Using a door for arms and back

Upper-body training in your office is fun because there are so many different exercises to choose from. Do a set of 10 repetitions and then write that important memo. During your next set, ponder a company takeover. The great thing is that you won't sweat bullets because you are cooling down between sets, writing memos, and answering the phone. Your creativity will improve when you add mini-workouts to your day. Your colleagues will marvel at your always-pumped, well-defined arms.

Treat your office workouts just as you would your gym workouts. Your chest muscles don't care whether they are pressing a bar or a desk. Train each upper-body muscle group no more than twice a week, but if you enjoy working out daily, split up your body parts. On Monday, train your chest and the backs of your arms. On Tuesday, work your back, shoulders, and the fronts of your arms. You could even tone a single muscle group each day.

Use perfect posture on every exercise. Hold your head up, shoulders back, stomach in, and chest out. Perform 10 repetitions of each exercise. Be careful not to lock your elbows. Begin each movement by drawing your navel in toward your spine using your lower-abdominal muscles. Continue to flex those muscles through the duration of your reps. Breathe normally or exhale on the exertion of each rep.

Push-Ups Off Your Desk

Push-Ups Off Your Desk are great for your chest, the backs of your arms, and shoulders. Make sure your desk is secured to the floor!

Performing desk push-ups is less challenging than doing them from the floor, so you may have to do several sets to fatigue your muscles. Draw an imaginary line from the top of your head to the back of your heel. Keep your wrist neutral and don't allow your back to sag.

YOUR PERSONAL TRAINER

Don't baby yourself during your office workouts. Your muscles don't know whether stimulation comes from a weight machine or pressing against the back of your chair.

Move slowly through each repetition—three seconds down, three seconds up. If it is too difficult to do a regular desk push-up, just bend your elbows a couple inches on each rep. As you get stronger, increase your range of motion. Never go beyond a 90-degree angle with your elbows. After a few months, you can challenge yourself further by stopping for three seconds every inch on your repetition down and every inch on your repetition up.

1. Stand about a foot away from your desk and place your hands shoulder-width apart on the top edge of your desk.

2. Lead with your chest as you lower your body toward the desk by bending your elbows.

3. When your elbows bend to 90 degrees, press back into your original position.

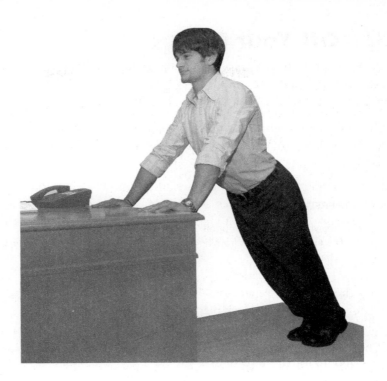

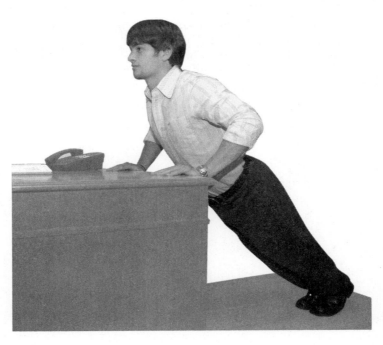

Dips Off Your Desk

Dips Off Your Desk tighten the backs of your arms, shoulders, and chest. Make sure that your desk is secured to the floor. Sit on the edge of your desk or chair and (as soon as no one's watching) begin your repetitions.

Maintain perfect posture throughout the duration of the exercise. At first, bend your elbows an inch or two on each repetition. You may rest in the up position if you need to. Use your legs to help you move up and down.

As you become stronger, bend your elbows a little more. Be careful not to bend your elbows farther than 90 degrees. Move slowly through each repetition. Breathe normally or exhale on the exertion phase of each rep. As you become more advanced, do not rest in the up or the down position and do not use your legs to help complete your reps.

IN OTHER WORDS

Your triceps consist of three muscles in the back of your arm. These muscles are used to extend your elbow for pushing movements.

1. Stand with your back to your desk and your hands placed behind you on your desk with your fingers pointed forward.

2. Use your legs for balance as you lower yourself by bending your elbows.

3. Extend your elbows and return to your starting position.

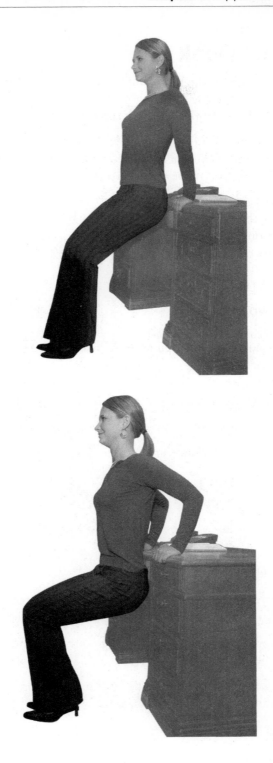

Squeeze the Desk

Squeeze the Desk firms the muscles in your chest. At first do not squeeze hard. Press with the palms and heels of your hands. Focus on your chest muscles flexing. As you get stronger, you may press harder.

Be sure to breathe normally while you are doing this exercise. Do not hold your breath. If you prefer, you may exhale through each repetition. If holding each repetition for three seconds is too challenging, begin with one second. Add a second a week until you can hold your desk press for three seconds.

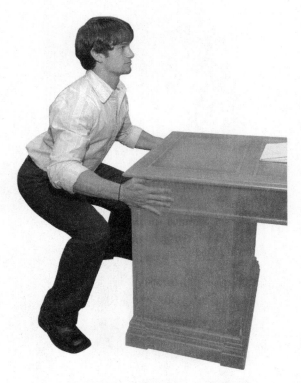

1. Face the narrow part of your desk. Place both palms on the outside of your desk with your elbows bent.

2. Press your palms into the desk, flexing your chest muscles. Hold for three seconds. Then relax.

3. Be sure to keep your back straight whether you squat down by bending your knees or lean over hinging at your hips.

Shoulder Flexion

Shoulder Flexion firms and tones the fronts of your shoulders. Perform this exercise either sitting or standing. Try this move from different angles so that you will firm and tone all parts of the fronts of your shoulders. For example, moving from a seated to a standing position changes the angle of the exercise.

If you are performing the exercise with your left arm, place your right hand on your left shoulder and feel the muscle flex. Be sure to breathe normally through the entire movement. If you prefer, you may exhale through each rep.

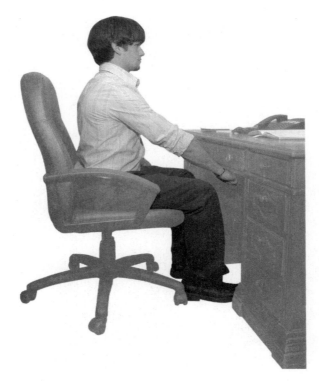

1. Sit in a military posture with the back of your right hand contacting the underside of your desk. (Keep your chest out, stomach in, shoulders back, and your head up.) Keep your elbow slightly bent.

2. Flex the front of your shoulder, pressing the back of your hand into the desk as if you are trying to lift it. Hold for three seconds. Then relax.

Back Exercise

Back Exercise adds form to your upper back. Before you begin this exercise, try it without moving. Simply grab the bottom of your chair with both hands, keep your back straight, and pull gently. You should feel the muscles in your back flex. These are the muscles you will be using to perform this exercise.

GET IT RIGHT

Be sure you maintain a balance between the musculature of the fronts of your arms and the backs of your arms to promote symmetry and prevent injury.

Be sure to breathe normally through the duration or, if you prefer, you may exhale through each rep. Use your arms as if they were hooks so that they do not fatigue. On the way up, you are training your back. On the way down, you are training both your abs and your back. Keep your neck relaxed throughout.

1. Grab the underside of your chair with your hands. While seated in your chair, pull your stomach in, and bend forward with your back straight, hinging from your hips.

2. Hold on to the underside of your chair as you extend your back to your original position.

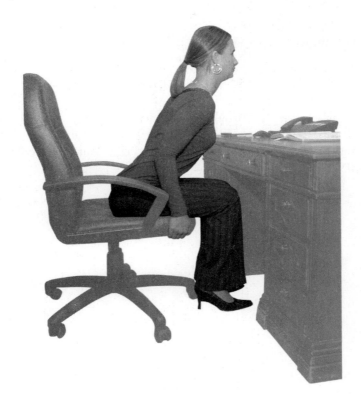

Doorknob Pull-Ups

Doorknob Pull-Ups firm your arms and back. This is a great full-body exercise because all of your muscles take part in the movement. Even your forearms get a great workout from gripping the doorknob.

As the muscles in your arms and back begin to fatigue, allow your legs to help you through each rep. As a further challenge, after you have completed your 10 reps, allow your legs to push you up into the start position, but on the way down use your arms and back to slow your descent. Be sure to use your legs for balance.

(Don't let your colleagues catch you doing this exercise or it will be very difficult to explain!)

1. Grab one doorknob in each hand.

2. Using your legs for balance, sink toward the floor as your arms extend.

3. Pull yourself back up. Use your legs if necessary.

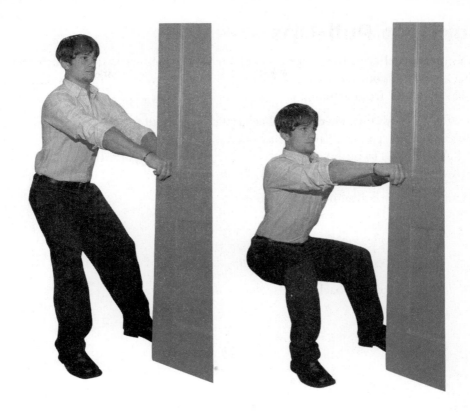

The Least You Need to Know

- A solid desk, a chair, and a door are all you need to do upper-body exercises at the office.
- Move slowly through your reps to gain maximum benefit.
- Desk sit-ups and dips are easy to do throughout the day.
- Exercise breaks at the office can help clear your head.

Upper Body at the Gym

In This Chapter

- Performing the king of upper-body exercises
- Targeting your arms and shoulders
- Working your back

The gym is a virtual paradise if you want to cut and define your upper body. With so many exercises and machines to choose from, you almost can't go wrong. But you *can* go wrong if you train too hard, too much, or with improper form.

Maintain perfect posture on all of your upper-body exercises. When in doubt, assume the military "attention" position. Keep your elbows slightly bent on all exercises. Never bring a bar behind your neck. Move slowly through each exercise so that you could stop at any given moment if necessary. Focus on the muscle group you're training and allow all your other muscles to relax. Be sure the amount of weight you use doesn't hurt your form.

If you begin to lose your form, stop the exercise immediately. If your muscles are sore from a previous workout, train a different body part. Move through a full range of motion on each exercise. Begin each exercise by using your lower abdominals to draw your navel into your spine. Exhale during the exertion phase of each rep.

Bench Press

The Bench Press focuses on your chest and the backs of your arms—it's the king of all upper-body exercises. Although gym rats may ask you how much you can bench, a more important question might be, "How do your chest and the backs of your arms look?"

Keep your thumbs under the bar and press your hands toward each other to keep your chest muscles flexed throughout the lift. When you lower the bar toward your chest, pause when your elbows are parallel to the floor and then exhale as you press the bar up. The bar will find its own path to the top of the range of motion, and it is generally not straight up and down. Your body naturally finds angles where your body is stronger. You can lift heavier weight with free weights where you can alter the angle of your lift. When you try to lift the same amount of weight on a machine that does not allow you to vary the angle of your lift, it will feel 10 pounds heavier.

After you press the weight up to the top, squeeze your chest muscles together as if you are trying to hold a nickel between them. Flex the backs of your arms, too.

1. Lie down with your back on the bench and your hands holding the weights shoulder-width apart. Squeeze your shoulder blades together in preparation for your lift.

2. Bend your elbows as you control the weight, slowly inching down until your elbows are parallel to the floor.

3. Slowly extend your elbows, returning to your starting position.

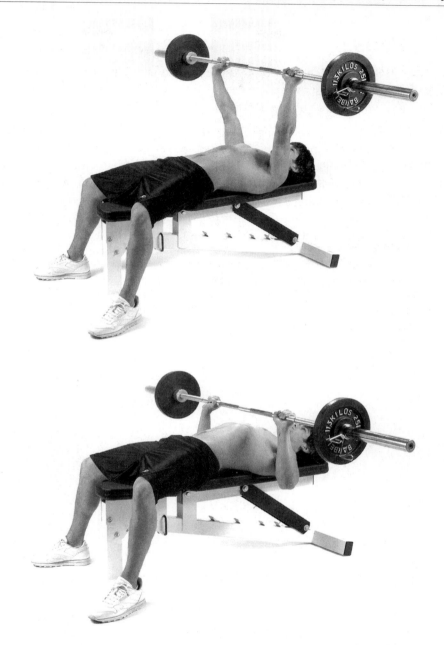

Triceps Press

The Triceps Press firms the backs of your arms. In fact, any exercise where you extend your elbows trains your triceps, so if this exercise doesn't meet your needs, find another angle where you are extending your elbows.

The main part of this exercise that tones your triceps is the last few inches just before you reach full extension on the up phase. Do not fully lock your elbows, but move to a position as close to lockout as possible. The only joints that should be moving are your elbows, to isolate the triceps and prevent other muscles from helping. Do not bend your elbows past 90 degrees on the down phase.

GET IT RIGHT

To protect your shoulders on the bench press, lighten the weight and never let your elbows drop lower than parallel to the floor.

1. Lie down on your back and hold the weights above your chest with your elbows almost fully extended.

2. Lower the weights toward your forehead very slowly until your elbows bend at 90 degrees.

3. Extend your elbows back to your starting position.

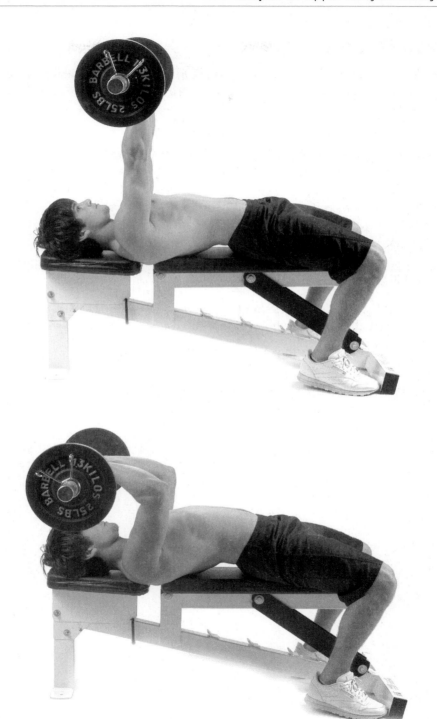

Lat Pull-Down

The Lat Pull-Down widens your upper back to create that "V" shape. Lead with your elbows and keep your body still. You may use either an overhand or underhand grip.

IN OTHER WORDS

Your latissimus dorsi is your upper-back muscle. There is no truth to the myth that if you use an extra-wide grip it widens your upper back even more.

The first movement you make should be to squeeze your shoulder blades together and press them down. Instead of jerking the bar, just by squeezing and depressing your shoulder blades you have stimulated activity in your lat muscles.

Resist the tendency to pull with your arms. Imagine your hands are hooks on the bar so that you do not squeeze too tightly.

1. Begin with your hands shoulder-width apart on the lat pull-down bar. Set the seat on the machine appropriately to avoid compromising your form.

2. Pull the bar down to your upper chest.

Maintain perfect form on the negative portion of this exercise by keeping your chest out and your back straight. Move very slowly and feel a full stretch on your lat muscle at the end of each rep.

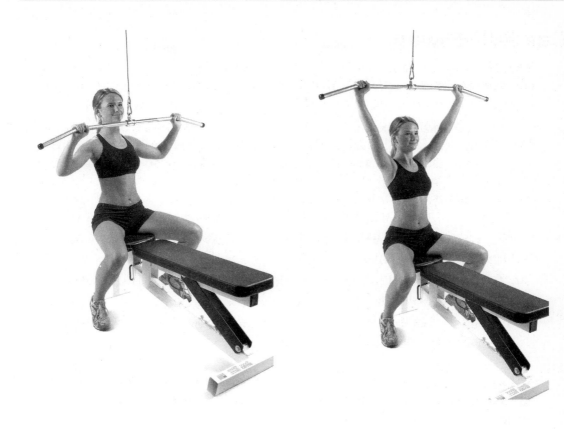

Seated Rowing

Seated Rowing firms the muscles of your middle back. These are the muscles between your shoulder blades. This is a very simple exercise, but you will see people in gyms make it very difficult and even dangerous.

The worst mistake you can make on this exercise is to lean forward or lean back. Even though it is called "Seated Rowing" most people tend to perform the exercise by leaning back or "rowing" rather than keeping their back straight. Keep your chest out as you pull the handles toward your chest. Keep your arms close to your sides so that your inner upper arm brushes by the side of your chest. Once again your hands are like hooks, so you don't use other muscles to jerk the weight forward.

At the completion of the movement, imagine the backs of your elbows as wings so that your elbows move toward each other.

1. Grab a handle with each hand with your elbows almost fully extended and your knees slightly bent.

2. Pull the handles toward your chest, keeping your elbows in close to your sides.

Allow the resistance to pull your hands back to the starting position until you feel a full stretch on your lats. Be sure to keep your chest out, stomach in, and back straight for the duration of all of your reps.

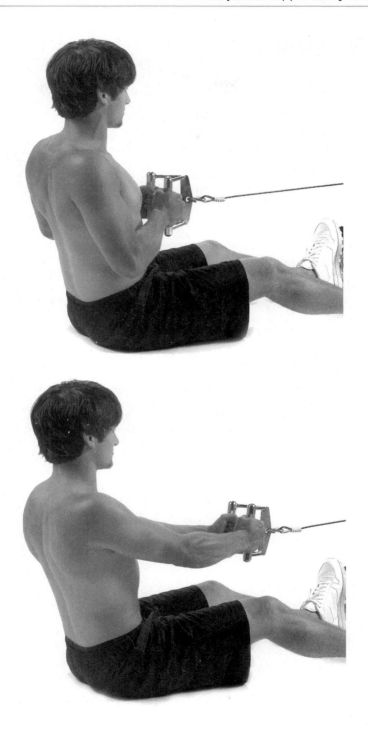

Shoulder Press

The Shoulder Press sculpts all three parts of your shoulder. Always press from the front of your neck instead of the back. You may perform this exercise seated or standing, but keep perfect posture throughout.

YOUR PERSONAL TRAINER

Strong muscles take over for weak or injured ones. Do not neglect your weaker muscles. If you don't use them, you'll lose them.

In the down position, your elbows should bend no further than 90 degrees. In the up position, extend your elbows until if pressed further, they would lock. Pause at the top. Flex the backs of your arms and lift your shoulders as if you were trying to touch your ears.

It doesn't matter whether you use barbells or dumbbells for this exercise. It is also your choice (if you use dumbbells instead of a straight bar) to either twist the elbows up into position or keep your palms facing forward.

1. Begin with the weights at shoulder level.

2. Extend your elbows over your head until they are almost straight.

3. Return your arms back to the starting position.

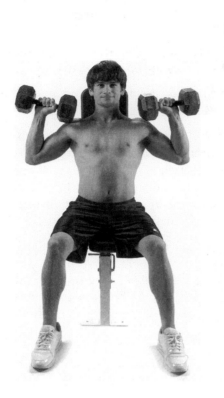
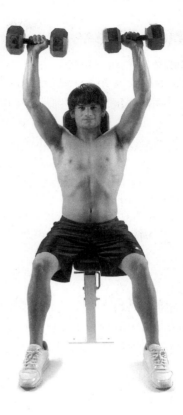

Biceps Curl

The Biceps Curl works the front of your upper arm. You may use a barbell or dumbbells for this exercise. Keep your body still during the entire exercise.

If you use dumbbells, you can perform this exercise either seated or standing. With a barbell you must stand throughout the exercise.

Move very slowly, because many people accidentally cheat on this exercise by bending the back and "kipping" the weight up. Another common mistake people make is to not go through the full range of motion, and cheat with half-reps. At the bottom of the rep, flex your triceps for a split second. Let your biceps do the work and you will see great results. Move slowly through both the up and the down phases, keeping constant tension on your biceps.

1. Begin in a standing position with your palms facing forward and the weights near your thighs with your elbows slightly bent.

2. Bend your elbows up slowly to a 45-degree angle.

3. Return to your starting position with the weights traveling the same path as on the upward pull.

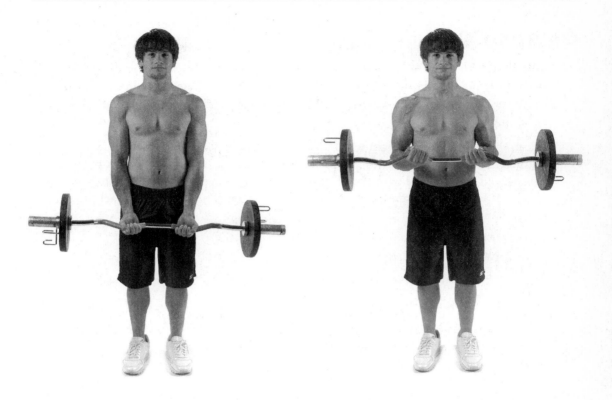

Reverse Curl

The Reverse Curl tones your forearms and the fronts of your upper arms. Press your feet firmly into the floor and resist the temptation to lean back, lift up on your toes, or move your feet. Keep your wrists in line with your forearms. Keep your elbows close to your body.

Be sure you use a light weight for this exercise. You may use an E-Z Curl bar, dumbbells, or a straight bar to complete this movement. Maintain perfect posture throughout the exercise with the elbows as the only moveable joint. Resist the temptation to swing the weight up into position. Keep your knees bent and back straight throughout.

BET YOU DIDN'T KNOW

Performing just 1 set of an exercise gives you 80 percent of the benefits of doing 3 sets.

1. Begin in a standing position with your palms facing backward and the weights near your thighs with your elbows slightly bent.

2. Bend your elbows up slowly to a 45-degree angle.

3. Return to your starting position with the weights traveling the same path.

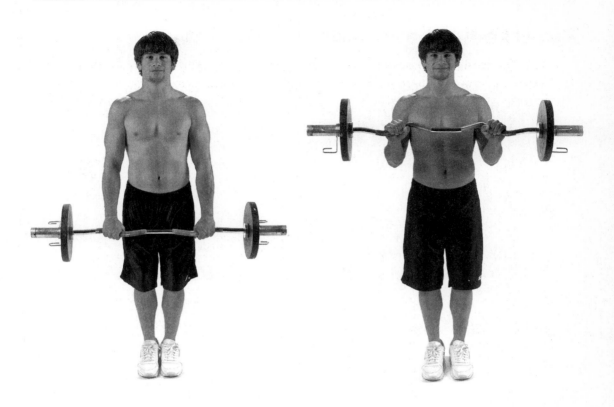

The Least You Need to Know

- The Bench Press works both the chest and the backs of the arms.
- Always keep your back straight when doing Seated Rowing.
- The Shoulder Press works all three muscles in the shoulder.
- Biceps and Reverse Curls work the front of the arms.

Shape and Sculpt

In This Chapter

- Combining workout time with TV time
- Pushing and pulling your way to results
- Learning the importance of variety
- Learning key upper-body stretches

This chapter shows you how to fit your upper-body workout into your busy life as well as proper stretching techniques. You don't need an expensive gym membership or equipment. You can train and stretch your upper body indoors, outdoors, or even while watching TV.

Your Favorite Sitcom Is Your Workout

It's easy to work out your upper body while watching your favorite TV shows. Push-ups are the greatest upper-body workout you can do during commercials. Begin in a push-up position on your hands and feet. Complete as many push-ups as possible.

As your arms and shoulders fatigue, drop to your knees until you cannot do another push-up. By then the commercial is over and you get to take a long break until your next set of push-ups.

The faster you move, the faster you will see definition and separation in your upper-body muscles. But start slowly and progress gradually. If you jump up and down as high as you can for a two-minute commercial you won't be able to get off the couch for your next bout of exercise. Walk, march, jog, and run, and eventually you might decide to jump.

BET YOU DIDN'T KNOW

A toned upper body means that your muscles are firing constantly. Keep those muscles firing by training consistently.

The Power of Two

The best bet for toning and defining your upper body without becoming fanatical is to combine pushing and pulling. All of the muscles in your chest, back, shoulders, and arms can be trained with variations of two exercises—pull-ups and push-ups.

To get a cardio workout and strengthen and tone every muscle in your upper body in a minimum amount of time, superset push-ups and pull-ups. Perform each set to failure. Failure simply means when you experience a break in your form:

- Cycle I is a set of wide grip pull-ups with an overhand grip. Then do a set of wide grip push-ups. Take a 30-second break.
- Cycle II is a set of close grip pull-ups with an underhand grip. Then do a set of close grip push-ups. Take a 30-second break.
- Cycle III is a set of shoulder-width grip pull-ups with an underhand grip. Then do a set of shoulder-width push-ups with your feet spread.

Don't be discouraged if you cannot do one push-up or pull-up. Moving quickly between sets and cycles keeps your heart rate up. Some people prefer pounding the pavement, but they don't get the muscular endurance and upper-body toning.

IN OTHER WORDS

You lose adipose tissue (fat) across your whole body over time. That is, you cannot lose fat on the back of your arm just by working your triceps.

Outdoor Training

If you have a yard, you don't need to spend hours in the gym. Use a push mower, and lawn mowing day becomes an upper-body workout.

YOUR PERSONAL TRAINER

The mode of training you choose should vary according to your time, energy level, and goals. This helps you attack your upper-body muscles at different angles and recruit more muscle fibers to enhance your training effect.

You can also get a great workout raking, gardening, and shoveling snow. You will be amazed at the intensity of your workout. Pushing, pulling, dragging, and cornering challenge your chest, back, shoulders, and arms at different angles better than the best celebrity infomercial exercise gizmo.

Mix It Up

Mix and match your exercise options and you will never get bored—but it's not just mental. If you do the same exercises day in and day out, you will get the same results. Soon, your muscles adapt and there will be no improvement.

Your upper body needs to be challenged or your muscles stagnate. Cross-training keeps you in great shape. Find a rock-climbing wall for Day One of your workout. Day Two you can swim. Day Three is cross-country skiing. And Day Four is an indoor elliptical machine with the upper-body option.

YOUR PERSONAL TRAINER

Stretch after your workout, not between sets of upper-body exercises. Stretching between sets makes you weaker for your next set.

Stretching Your Upper Body

Many of the strengthening exercises that you do for your upper body stretch your muscles at the end of your range of motion. For example, when you extend your elbows for your biceps curl, you stretch the fronts of your arms. The lat pull-down or pull-up stretches your back and chest.

However, it's a good idea for you to set aside a few minutes after each workout for stretching.

GET IT RIGHT

Hold your stretch instead of bouncing. Bouncing through your stretches may cause micro-tears in your muscles, damaging the fibers.

In fact, it's best to stretch at the completion of your workout to help prevent cramps and soreness. Warm up before you stretch. If you can find a warm room, that helps your muscles to relax and elongate. Relax into each stretch and concentrate on lengthening the belly of the muscle. Exhale as you move into each position. Learn to hold your stretch at least 10 seconds in order to fully relax the muscle. Add 2 seconds a week until you work up to 30 seconds. Within months you may stretch to a slight level of tension, but never approaching pain.

Triceps Stretch

The Triceps Stretch lengthens the back of your upper arm. Keep your back straight, shoulders down, and neck aligned with your back. Resist the temptation to drop your head forward. Flexible triceps are important for any throwing motion. Be careful not to bring your elbow back too far behind your head.

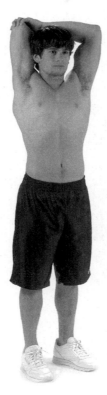

1. Stand with your feet shoulder-width apart and your knees slightly bent. Reach back with your right arm as if you were trying to scratch the middle of your back. Your right elbow is now beside your ear. Grab your elbow with your left hand.

2. Pull your elbow gently toward the ceiling until you feel a stretch.

3. Switch arms and repeat.

Shoulder Stretch

The Shoulder Stretch loosens up the muscles in your shoulder. Maintaining shoulder flexibility is important for just about every upper-body movement that you make.

Keep your shoulders parallel to the floor, your back straight, and your eyes looking over the horizon. Resist the temptation to twist your entire upper body.

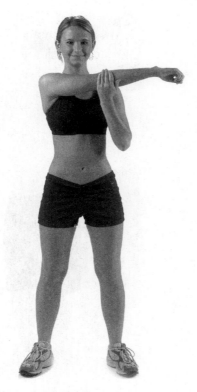

1. Stand with your feet shoulder-width apart and your knees slightly bent. Bring your right arm across your body so that your right elbow is in front of your chest.

2. Grab the back of your right upper arm with your left hand and gently pull to the left.

3. Switch arms and repeat.

Chest Stretch

The Chest Stretch lengthens the muscles in your upper, middle, and lower chest. Flexibility in your chest will maintain your posture. If your chest is tight, your shoulders roll forward into a slumping pattern.

Keep your shoulders parallel and down throughout this stretching exercise. Keep your chin up and your chest out.

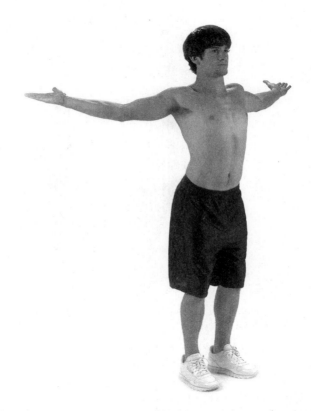

1. Stand with your feet shoulder-width apart and your knees slightly bent. Extend your arms out to the side with your palms facing up.

2. Flex the muscles in your middle back to pull your arms back. Hold when you feel the stretch in your chest.

Upper-Back Stretch

The Upper-Back Stretch lengthens the muscles in the upper part of your back. This is a "feel good" stretch. Bring your chin down to your chest and relax into the stretch. If you suffer from knee problems, do this exercise standing, while facing a wall.

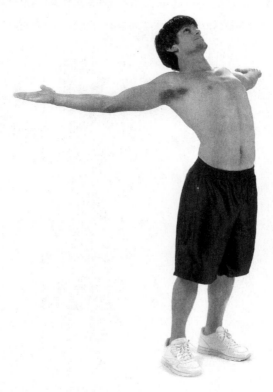

1. Move to the floor on your hands and knees. Bend your knees into a fully flexed position.

2. Keep your hands where they are so that when you bend your knees you feel a stretch in your upper back.

The Least You Need to Know

- Do push-ups during TV commercials.
- Combine different types of activities so the same muscles aren't worked all the time.
- Stretch at the end of your workout to prevent cramps and soreness.
- Incrementally work up to holding stretches for 30 seconds.

Abdominals

This part shows you how to work the four muscle groups in your abdomen—your internal and external obliques, your six-pack, and underneath it all your transverse abdominis. Stretches and exercises you can perform at home, the gym, and the office will help you firm up your stomach and love handles.

Abdominals Made Simple

In This Chapter

- The four muscle groups of abs
- The reason traditional sit-ups don't work
- The intercostals and serratus muscles
- The way back muscles play a role in ab work

The one muscle group that never goes out of style is your abdominals. Advertisers have hooked people into thinking that a tight midsection is the ultimate goal. Men size up other men by a quick glance at the size of their belly, and women certainly take notice as well. Popular magazines exhort women to banish their love handles and pooch.

It is important to begin working on your abdominals by understanding the anatomy and function of them so that you will better grasp the training concepts presented later. By understanding how each abdominal muscle functions and their location, you'll be able to work your abs efficiently, and firm and tone them to their full potential. There are four major muscle groups in the abdominal region, and a couple other eye-catching muscles in the surrounding area. Contrary to general thought, your abs aren't just in the front of your stomach. They are an amazing pattern of muscles connected to your hips, ribcage, and your backbone. To have great abs, you need to do belly exercises, lower-back moves, and side-of-your-stomach toners.

If you sit and stand with perfect posture, your lower pooch will all but disappear.

Your abs include four muscle groups:

1. Your six-pack or rectus abdominis

2. Your side abs or external obliques

3. Your internal obliques, underneath your side abs

4. Underneath all of these muscles, your transverse abdominis

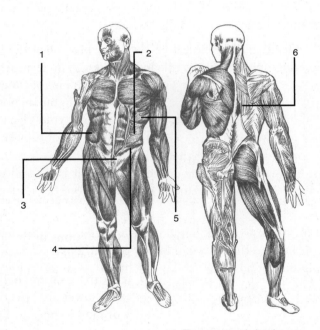

1. External oblique
2. Internal oblique
3. Rectus abdominis

4. Transverse abdominus
5. Serratus anterior
6. Erector spinae (back muscle group)

The muscle groups in your abdomen.

No Old-Fashioned Sit-Ups

Great care and excellent technique are required to strengthen the abdominal muscles. To be effective, you must pull your chest toward the knees using only the abdominal group. Often, however, other, more powerful muscles (those that flex the legs and hips) do much of the work.

Sounds like toning your stomach is a job for the good old sit-up you did in P.E. class. The problem with regular sit-ups is that you work every other muscle besides your abs. You pull on your neck, and your legs do most of the work because you have someone holding your ankles. Traditional sit-ups emphasize sitting up rather than pulling your chest toward your hips. Most people tend to compromise their form when reaching their fatigue level, and a common mistake people make is pulling on their neck when tired.

Sit-ups are inefficient because the hip flexor works best when the legs are straight as they are when doing sit-ups. The hip flexor muscle lies underneath your abs and connects the lower part of your spine to your upper leg. Its main function is to raise your leg in front of you. When you flex it, your leg raises. If you anchor your ankles for a sit-up, your hip flexor does most of the work in pulling your chest toward your knees. Worse than that, regular sit-ups grind the vertebrae in your lower back.

 GET IT RIGHT

To maintain your eye-catching abs, take the hip flexors out of your ab exercises.

Exercises presented in the home, office, and gym sections in the following chapters show you ways to take the hip flexors out of the equation.

Just as you can't contract half of your thigh, you can't contract half of your abs. There goes the notion of training your "upper abs" and "lower abs" in complete isolation. However, you can focus on the upper bundles of muscle fiber by moving just the torso or the lower fibers by moving the hips.

If you have well-defined upper abs and you can't see your lower abs, it's not that your lower abs need more work. It just means you've got fat covering them.

Your upper abs are stimulated when you do crunches without resistance, but when you add resistance the lower abs work equally as much. Reverse crunches work the lower abs more than the upper abs, but the obliques also help in that exercise. The lesson here is that when you add resistance to an abdominal exercise, all of your ab muscles join in to get the job done.

You might be afraid to add resistance to your ab exercises for fear of developing muscular love handles, but because the side-ab abdominal wall is a sheet of muscle, even if you add resistance to your side-ab exercises the muscle is unlikely to protrude. Your side-ab muscles don't have the capacity to expand like your front-ab muscles do. A large waist comes from a lot of fat in that area, a large pelvic girdle, or a beer belly.

Your Six-Pack

Your *rectus abdominis* is a wide, flat sheath of muscle, commonly referred to as your six-pack. It stretches from the bottom of the ribs down to just below the navel (belly button). The six-pack is not six muscles. It is visible sections of a single muscle. It is similar to your thigh muscle, but with partitions. The partitions are fibrous bands called tendinous inscriptions.

When you flex your rectus abdominis muscle to lean forward, your lower back bends about 30 degrees. The rectus abdominis is responsible for bending forward at the waist and drawing your pelvis upward.

These front stomach muscles pull your chest toward your hips. In essence, the main thing your front stomach muscles do is decrease the distance between your chest and hips.

Side Abs

A safe guess is that you want to cut and define your conductor muscle (your six-pack), but what about the orchestra (your side abs)? The conductor is only as good as the orchestra, and your six-pack would be better looking if you spent time developing the side abs as well.

Love handles are those rolls of fat that you can pinch on the sides of your waist. Your well-defined six-pack is adulterated by a matching set of love handles. But just beneath this layer of fluff is a powerful set of muscles called your *obliques.*

Although you cannot spot reduce your love handles, you can tone the oblique muscles underneath. Do this and your waistline will be firmer, flatter, and tighter. And when you shed the fat that surrounds them, your entire waistline will be cut and defined. Tone your obliques while whittling away your love handles. Love handles generally disappear in men when their percentage of body fat drops into the single digits. Women only have to get their body fat level down to about 15 percent.

External Obliques

Your *external obliques* are the muscles at the sides of the waist—the sexy muscles under your love handles. They form a "V" shape from the ribs down to below your navel. Tuck your fingers into your front pockets. That is the shape of your external obliques.

Your external obliques are used when you twist and bend forward. They are activated by twisting in your chair, or bending down to pick up that pen on the floor. Strong obliques help to pull, lift, or push heavy objects. Your obliques are the only abdominal muscles constantly active during standing. They function while you are in an upright posture to brace your torso. Together, these muscles contract to tilt the torso, as well as twist it, from side to side. They steady your torso to keep gravity from pulling you out of balance.

Your external obliques help with your crunches and they brace your spine. Your oblique muscles are interwoven all the way around your middle. This provides lower-back support when you move. If the waist moves, the external obliques are involved. The torso rotation in golf and tennis is mostly done by the external obliques.

Even the basic crunch motion wouldn't be possible without a strong, flexed set of external obliques to steady your torso. Well-developed obliques make your waist tighter.

 BET YOU DIDN'T KNOW

The external obliques are the largest of the abdominal muscles.

Internal Obliques

Your *internal obliques* are underneath your external obliques. They extend diagonally down the sides of your waist forming an inverted "V" from your pelvis to your lower ribs. Your internal obliques run in the opposite direction of your external obliques.

Your obliques are thin muscles. They are not designed for heavy resistance training. They enclose your organs. Similar to the externals, the internal obliques are involved in torso rotation. You also use these muscles when you breathe deeply. Both the internal and external obliques are responsible for the twisting movement of your torso and side bends. For your torso to twist, your internal oblique and the opposite external oblique flex. If you wanted to bend to one side, both the internal and external obliques on the same side flex simultaneously. That is why "oblique twists" work well to train these muscles. When you do these exercises, curl your trunk forward and diagonally so that your left armpit moves toward your right hip.

A great toning exercise for these muscles is the side plank. Another exercise that uses the rotating capabilities of your internal obliques is the "scissors." Your obliques are used in almost every move you make, so train them well.

Although your obliques are not designed to grow huge no matter how hard you train them, keep them strong to maintain ideal postural alignment.

GET IT RIGHT

If you happen to be one of the unfortunate genetically gifted few whose sides grow larger from oblique work, then minimize your oblique training.

Transverse Abdominis

The *transverse abdominis* (TVA) muscle lies beneath all of your other abdominal muscles, and therefore cannot be felt with your hands nor can it be seen. It's a thin muscle that runs horizontally, surrounding your abdomen.

Although this muscle is invisible, your TVA is responsible for keeping your waist nicely tucked in. When you suck in your stomach to look skinny, you are using your TVA. You can feel it flex when you cough or sneeze. Think of it as a girdle because it functions as a compressor for the abdomen, keeping everything in place. It contracts when the other ab muscles are working. The TVA does not bend your spine. It serves as a brace for your lower back.

BET YOU DIDN'T KNOW

The *kiai* in karate trains your TVA. So does the forceful breathing of Lamaze.

Training your TVA is easy. From the beginning position of any ab exercise, exhale slowly and use your abs to gently draw in the sides of your torso as you bring your lower ribs toward your hips. Bring your navel as close as possible to your spine.

Imagine you're wearing a girdle or weight-lifting belt. Pull it tight. Now tighten it another notch. This is your TVA in action, creating the appearance of a smaller waist. Train this muscle daily, and your TVA (and obliques) will be the only weight-lifting belt that you will ever need. But activating your TVA takes concentration and practice.

Intercostals

The *intercostals* are the breathing muscles that lie between your ribs. They are bands of muscle angling downward in the sides of the ribcage and the upper abdomen. The intercostals flex the torso and cause it to twist, so doing any type of elbow-to-opposite-knee exercise will stimulate this group of muscles.

Serratus

The serratus anterior muscles are the fingerlike strands of muscle on the ribcage between the front abs and the lats. You can feel them flex when you attempt to lower your ribcage.

Your serratus muscles make your upper body look more defined when you have little *subcutaneous fat.* The serratus helps when you push heavy objects off your chest at various angles, controls the separation of your shoulder blades, and assists in lifting your shoulders. If you're very lean and muscular, your serratus and external obliques form a criss-cross of muscular definition. The "fingers to toes" exercise trains your serratus.

IN OTHER WORDS

Subcutaneous fat is the adipose tissue between your skin and ab muscles that smoothes out definition.

Back Muscles

Back muscles co-contract with your ab muscles to perform the exercises in this program. The back muscles are called the *erector spinae*, and they run the entire length of your spine on either side of your vertebrae. They bend your spine backward and sideways and act as a brace.

Your back muscles also counterbalance your movement when your abs flex and you lean forward. No abs program is complete without training your back: strong abs equal a strong back, and vice versa. If you ignore your back while strengthening your abdominals, you encourage and promote poor posture. That's why this book has several exercises that train your abs and back simultaneously. Exercises such as squats, dead lifts, and the bench press tax the abs as stabilizers better than almost anything else, when performed with enough intensity.

Strong pelvic floor muscles are crucial to a strong back. When you contract the pelvic floor muscles (by doing a kegal exercise) at the same time as you contract your transverse abdominis, other deep muscles in your back are activated. These muscles are directly responsible for bracing your spine during your ab training.

Firm, tight abs make you look and feel better. Every time you move, your abs are involved. In the following chapters, you will learn exercises that you can perform at home, at work, or while waiting in line. Don't wait. You can begin your training right now while reading this paragraph. Simply exhale and contract your abs by bringing your lower back flat into your chair. Read the rest of this book and you can get the abs you've always dreamed of.

The Least You Need to Know

- Adding resistance helps work all of your ab muscles.
- The side plank exercise tones the inner obliques.
- Strengthen your back as well as your abs to prevent poor posture.
- Traditional sit-ups don't work your abs; do crunches instead.

Abs at Home

In This Chapter

- Proper form for ab exercises
- Crunch your six-pack into shape
- Exercises that target each ab muscle
- The way to eliminate love handles

When you're talking about your midsection, you want less flab and more muscle. Men want their abs rock-hard, ripped, and defined, while women prefer them to be sleek, tight, and flat. Men want to lose their love handles and women will gladly give away their pooch. Unfortunately, men generally carry extra fat around the waist and women have to deal with the pooch.

This chapter takes you through your home ab-isolation program. Do these exercises in street clothes—no need to change. Each exercise only takes 30 seconds. Do 10 repetitions of each exercise. Maintain perfect posture and exhale on the exertion portion of each exercise. Move slowly through each repetition—three seconds up, three seconds down. Never sacrifice your form by trying to get in a few extra reps. Add 2 repetitions per week until you can perform 20 consecutive repetitions.

Posture Perfect

Maintain perfect posture and you demonstrate confidence and a balance between your abs and back. Contract your stomach muscles by bringing your navel toward your spine. Imagine a piece of string tied around your waist. If you allow your belly to bulge, the string will break. This is one of the best exercises for making that lower pooch disappear.

YOUR PERSONAL TRAINER

Whether exercising, standing in line, or sitting at your computer, maintaining perfect posture is a great ab exercise.

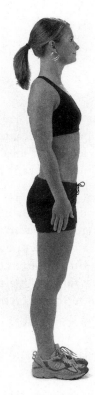

1. Keep your head up, shoulders back, and stomach in.

2. Don't hide your abs; keep your back straight.

Perfect Crunch

Perform the Perfect Crunch and you firm and tone those eye-catching muscles in the front of your stomach. The crunch is the best exercise for targeting all of your abdominal muscles at the same time. Just before you start your crunch, pretend someone is about to hit you in the stomach. Feel your stomach muscles contract and keep using them throughout the duration of your reps.

Bring your ribs toward your hips on each rep. Exhale on each rep and draw your navel in toward your spine. Keep your neck in the same position throughout each repetition. Imagine an apple between your chin and your chest. Do not put your hands behind your neck. You will be tempted to start pulling at your neck to get the last few reps, which places unnecessary strain on this fragile part of the spine.

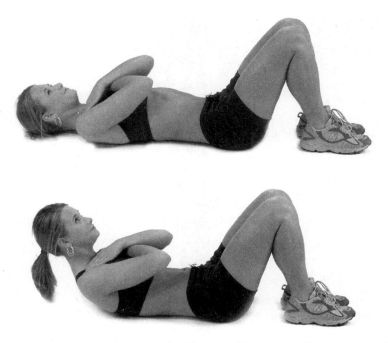

1. Flatten your lower back to the floor and bend your knees to 90 degrees with your feet flat on the floor.

2. Fold your arms across your chest.

3. As you exhale your breath, curl your chest a couple inches off of the floor.

4. Hold, then slowly lower your back to the floor and continue your reps.

Pulsing

Pulsing is a continuous exercise that trains your front ab muscles without resting between reps. Keep your abs flexed for the entire set. Your fingers should rest behind your head. They stay open but they do not touch each other. When you interlock your fingers, you inadvertently pull on your head. If this exercise is too difficult, cross your arms in front of your chest. If crossing your arms over your chest is too challenging, bring your arms to your side. Exhale through pursed lips during each abbreviated rep.

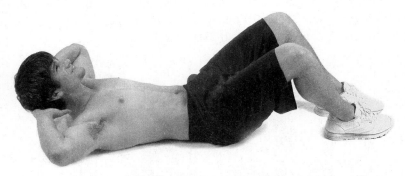

1. Lie on your back with your knees bent and your fingers resting behind your head.

2. Bring your chest toward your knees so that your shoulder blades are just a few inches from the floor.

3. Move about an inch in either direction, pulsing up and down.

GET IT RIGHT

Your rectus abdominis (six-pack) on the front of your stomach is a single muscle. If you train your lower abs, your upper abs are working, too.

Fingers to Toes

Fingers to Toes tones the front of your abs with particular concentration on your upper-ab muscles. It also targets those fingerlike muscles around your ribs. Keep your neck relaxed and don't try to reach too far. If you can keep your hips off of the floor, you'll increase the intensity of the exercise. Exhale during the up phase of each rep as you pull your navel toward your spine. Begin the movement from your abs and not your arms.

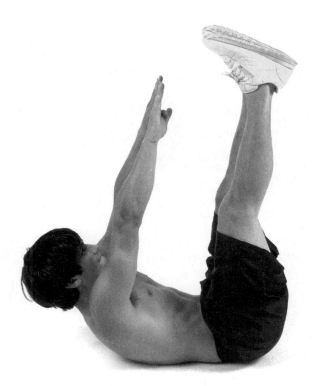

1. Lie on your back with your feet pointed toward the ceiling and your knees straight.

2. Hinge from your waist and extend your fingers toward your toes, and raise your hips off of the floor. Keep your back flat to the floor.

3. Lower your hips and shoulders back to the floor.

Reverse Crunch

The Reverse Crunch trains the muscles below your naval. Women call this area the pooch—the baby pooch. Firming the muscles in this area helps you to stand taller. Be sure your hips come off of the floor during each repetition. Keep your head and neck resting comfortably on the floor for the entire exercise. Exhale during the up phase of each rep and pull your navel in toward your spine. Maintain a smooth, rolling motion for both the up and the down phase. Keep your knees together for the entire exercise. Stop immediately if you have a break in your form.

GET IT RIGHT

When you train beyond "the burn," you set yourself up for injury.

1. Lie on your back with your knees bent and your feet flat on the floor.

2. Keep your arms by your sides.

3. Slowly bring your knees toward your chest until your hips come off the floor.

4. Move your knees back until your feet are about an inch from the floor.

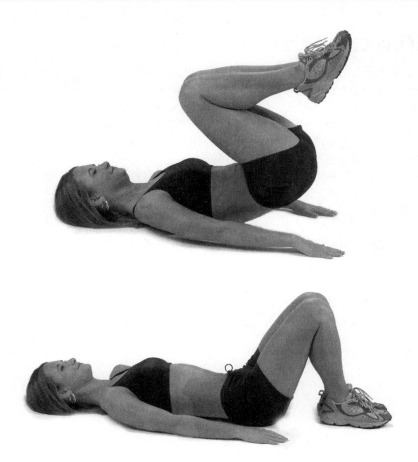

Scissors

Scissors is an exercise for the lower abs and side abs. If you had to choose one exercise besides crunches to target your entire abdominal area, this is the one. Your lower back remains on the floor. Exhale through pursed lips on each rep. Draw your navel in toward your spine. Your elbow moves toward your opposite knee and your knee moves toward your opposite elbow in a smooth, reciprocal motion. Maintain flexed abs through the duration of the movement. Keep your hands relaxed (do not pull with your hands) so that your neck doesn't bend forward. When fatigue sets in, be careful not to twist your neck back and forth. If you have a break in your form, stop immediately.

BET YOU DIDN'T KNOW

The reason we suggest you keep your back flat to the floor and do not recommend maintaining your natural lower back curve is that you might arch your back too much and strain yourself.

1. Lie on your back with your fingers resting behind your head.

2. Raise your right knee and touch it to your left elbow.

3. Raise your left knee and touch it to your right elbow.

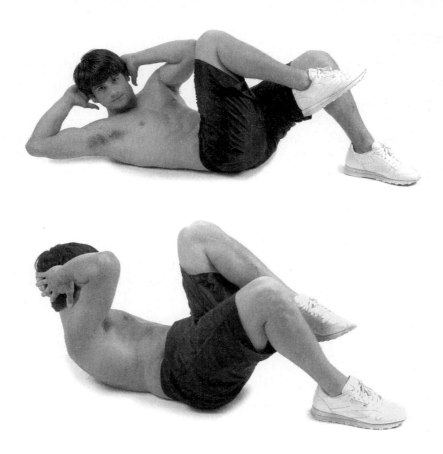

Knee-Ups

Knee-Ups are an advanced exercise for your lower abs, almost like a reverse crunch from a vertical position. Because your lower body is working against gravity, this is considered a very advanced exercise. Keep your shoulders down, neck relaxed, and head and chest up. Round your back and follow through with your hips so your abs are doing the work. Exhale on each rep and draw your navel in toward your spine. Resist the temptation to swing back and forth. Move very slowly, minimizing momentum. If this exercise is too difficult, try raising one knee at a time.

GET IT RIGHT

Train your abs like any other muscle group. Give them at least a day's rest before training them again.

1. Brace yourself between two chairs, elbows slightly bent.

2. Raise your knees toward your chest.

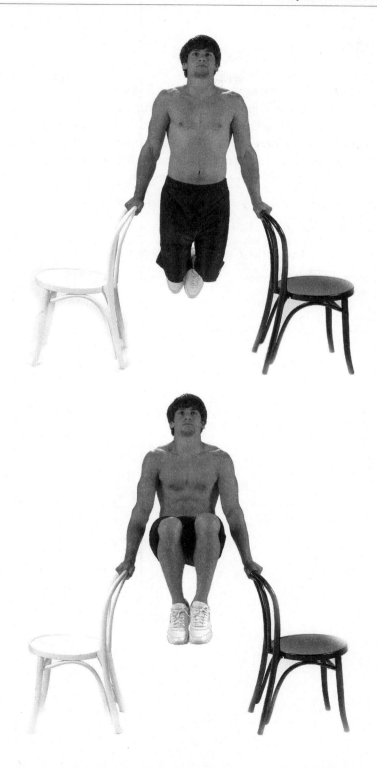

Leg Swings

Leg Swings train the side of your stomach. This is an advanced exercise. The straighter you keep your knees, the harder the exercise. Bend your knees as much as you need to when you first begin doing leg swings. Exhale on each rep and draw your navel in toward your spine. Keep your head and neck relaxed. All movement should begin from your abs. To increase the intensity, pause for a second at the bottom of each rep. If you feel any lower-back pain, substitute another side-ab exercise for this one.

1. Lie on your back with your arms out to your sides.

2. Raise your feet toward the ceiling.

3. Lower your legs to the right until they are 5 inches from the floor.

4. Repeat on your left side.

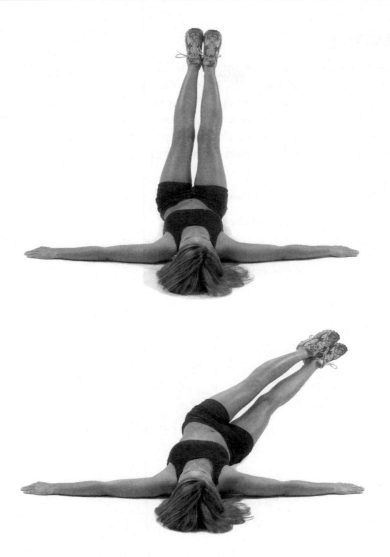

Side Ab-Ups

Side Ab-Ups target the muscles on the sides of your stomach. You may either alternate sides on each repetition or do all of your reps on one side and then all of your reps on the other side. Begin each repetition by flexing your abs. Rest between repetitions if necessary. Keep your neck relaxed. Exhale on each rep and draw your navel in toward your spine. To increase the intensity, bring your fingertips behind your head while your elbows remain out to the side. If this exercise is too difficult, reach your hand toward your opposite knee.

1. Lie on your back with your knees bent.

2. Cross your arms across your chest.

3. Lift your right shoulder toward your left knee.

4. Lift your left shoulder toward your right knee.

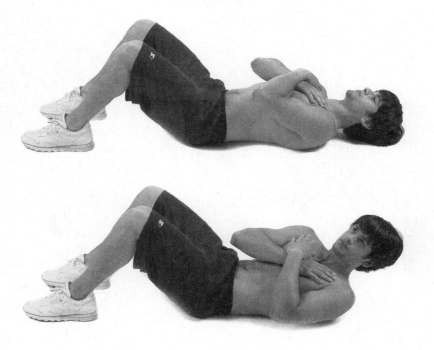

YOUR PERSONAL TRAINER

Because you probably do not want the rectus abdominis muscles (six-pack) underneath your waistline to grow larger, there is no need to overtrain your abs.

Inside Side Abs Reach

The Inside Side Abs Reach trains muscles on the sides of your stomach and the muscles underneath them. Exhale on each rep and draw your navel in toward your spine. Your head and neck should remain aligned. Although you can't see some of the muscles that are working underneath, they keep your stomach in when you maintain your posture. Don't try to bend too far in either direction when you do this exercise.

1. Lie on your back with your arms to your sides.

2. Slide your right hand toward your right foot.

3. Switch sides and repeat.

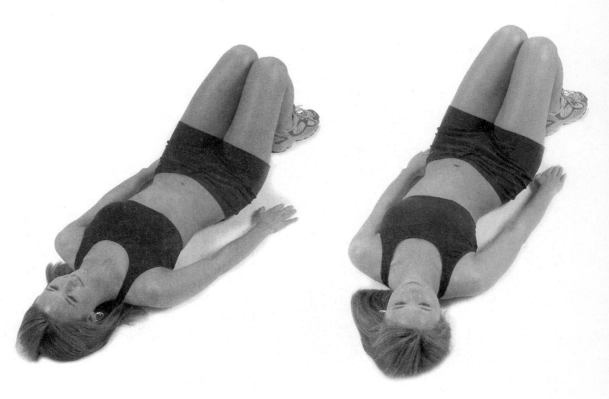

The Least You Need to Know

- Don't support your neck during crunches to avoid straining it.
- The Reverse Crunch helps firm up "the pooch" below the navel.
- Scissors is a great exercise for lower and side abs.
- Knee-Ups and Leg Swings are advanced ab exercises and may take practice to achieve.

Abs at the Office

In This Chapter

- Tone your abs while on the phone
- Ab exercises without motion
- Ab-toning chair and desk workouts

You will be amazed by the results you can achieve by performing simple ab exercises at the privacy of your desk. It's not about sets and reps. You don't need barbells and dumbbells to train your abs. Between phone calls, try the Abs at the Office routine. Flex your abs while typing on your computer or retrieving your messages.

Hold each movement for three seconds. Begin each exercise by drawing your navel into your spine. Be sure to breathe through each exercise instead of holding your breath. Maintain perfect posture, keeping your neck relaxed, chest out, and stomach in. Don't push too hard.

Chair Exercise—Upper Abs

The Chair Exercise—Upper Abs trains your upper-stomach muscles. You may do this exercise while talking on the phone or contemplating a decision. Because your abdominal muscles are endurance muscles, do this exercise several times a day, whenever the mood strikes. While you are leaning back, keep your neck in line with your back. Keep your chin up and don't look down toward your chest. Imagine an apple tucked between your chin and your chest.

If this exercise is too difficult, don't lean back all the way to the chair. Instead, lean back until you feel your abs flex. To further tone your abs, cross your arms over your chest. And to make this exercise more challenging, place your fingers behind your head in the "TV position." Never interlock your fingers or pull on your head with your hands. Keep your back straight and your head centered directly over your shoulders.

IN OTHER WORDS

A static contraction is when you squeeze your stomach muscles by holding them flexed without moving.

1. Sit on the edge of your chair with your arms extended to the front.

2. Contract your abs and lean back slowly until your upper back touches the back of your chair.

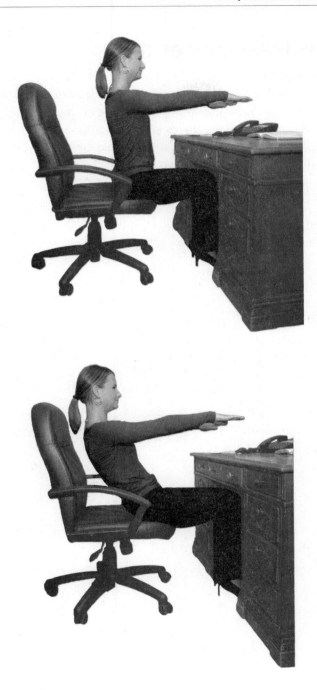

Using Your Desk—Front Abs

Using Your Desk—Front Abs trains the front of your stomach. This exercise strengthens the front abs as well as the top of your leg muscles. Stand up and stretch your legs between sets. Be careful not to press longer than three seconds and don't press too hard. Keep your shoulders back and head up. You may have a tendency to hold your breath during this exercise, so remember to breathe normally. You may also exhale during the exertion phase of each repetition if you prefer. Gradually increase the intensity of each static contraction as you get stronger.

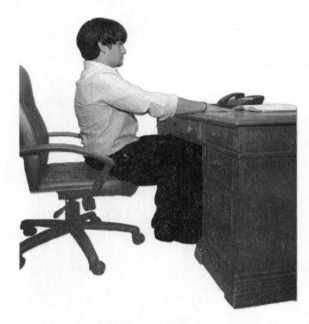

1. Sit in the front of your chair and lift your knees so that they are pressing against the underside of your desk.

2. Place your hands on top of the desk for balance and contract your abs for three seconds, then relax.

Chair Exercise—Front Abs

The Chair Exercise—Front Abs trains the front of your stomach. If you enjoy this exercise, consider trying out for the gymnastics team. Gymnasts have awesome abs and this exercise is one of the reasons why. At first, press your forearms into the chair and un-weight your hips from the chair. Keep your knees bent when performing this exercise. No one should detect you are exercising. As your abs get stronger, you may actually be able to lift your hips off of the chair. To challenge yourself further, extend your knees into an "L-Seat." When you can perform an L-Seat, show your colleagues and they will be impressed. Keep your back straight and exhale on each repetition.

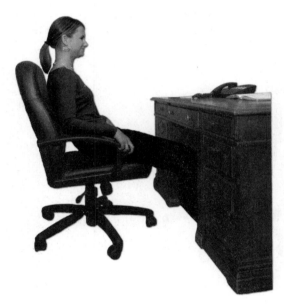

1. Sit in your chair with your back straight and your forearms placed securely on your armrests.

2. Press your forearms into the chair; contract your stomach muscles as if you are lightening the pressure on your seat.

YOUR PERSONAL TRAINER

Train your stomach muscles at different angles if you want to see great results.

Chair Exercise—Curls with Resistance

The Chair Exercise—Curls with Resistance trains the front of your stomach and your back. Keep your neck relaxed and your eyes forward. Your arms should remain bent and act as hooks so that they do not fatigue. Flex your abs on the way down and squeeze your abs and back muscles on the way up. Be sure to breathe normally and pay particular attention to your posture. You may exhale on the down phase if you prefer. To make this exercise challenging, add more resistance from your arms.

1. Grab underneath your thighs with both hands and curl your chest toward your legs.

2. Use your arms as resistance as you bring your chest back into your original position.

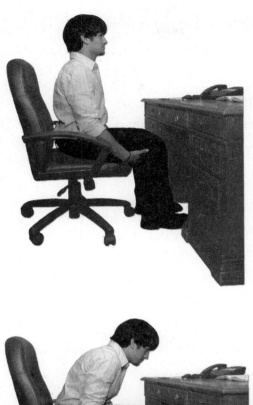

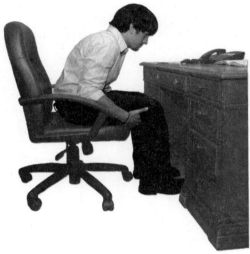

Chair Exercise—Lower Abs

The Chair Exercise—Lower Abs trains the lower part of your stomach. Be sure to brace your upper body by grabbing the armrests for balance. Raise your feet an inch off of the floor for one second. To add intensity, raise your feet a couple inches and hold for two seconds. Three inches and three seconds is a very challenging goal to shoot for. If this exercise is too difficult, raise one leg at a time. At first, alternate legs. Then perform all of your reps with one leg, and then all of your reps with the other. This is a very difficult exercise, so start slowly and progress gradually.

The difference between this exercise and Using Your Desk—Front Abs is that on that one you press against the desk as resistance. In Chair Exercise—Lower Abs, the resistance is the weight of your legs, but rather than pressing against the desk you attempt to lift your knees higher than you do on Using Your Desk—Front Abs. This extra range of motion increases the intensity of the exercise.

1. Sit with perfect posture on the front edge of your chair with your back straight and your neck relaxed.

2. Raise your knees toward your chest and then slowly lower them back to the floor.

BET YOU DIDN'T KNOW

On most stomach exercises, it is very difficult to isolate a certain muscle. All of them work together to get the job done.

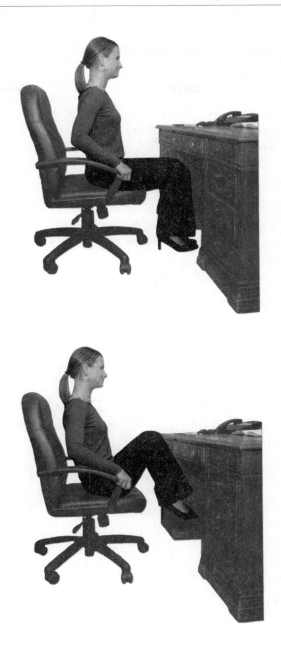

Chair Exercise—Side Abs

The Chair Exercise—Side Abs trains the sides of your stomach. Keep your shoulders down and your chest out. The first movement you make is to flex the right side of your stomach closest to your right armrest. Do not lean more than a couple inches, and think of it as tilting your body sideways from your waist instead of bending forward. If you perform it correctly, your office mates shouldn't notice you're doing this exercise.

Keep your neck relaxed and breathe normally or exhale on each rep if you prefer. At first, alternate sides with each rep. To make the exercise more challenging, perform all of your reps on one side and then do all of your reps on the other side.

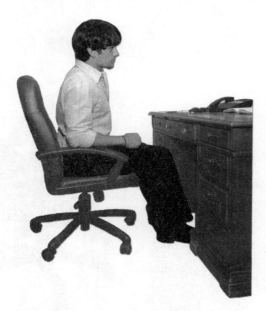

1. Place your right forearm on the armrest and flex the right side of your stomach. Hold for three seconds.

2. Switch sides and repeat.

Chair Exercise—Advanced Side Abs

The Chair Exercise—Advanced Side Abs exercise trains the muscles on the sides of your stomach. Be sure to twist your upper body in the direction of the knee you are lifting. Your knee doesn't have to contact your elbow, so don't bend over more than a couple inches from your waist. If this exercise is too difficult, bring your hand toward the opposite knee instead of the elbow.

To challenge yourself further on this exercise, place your fingers behind your head and bring your knee toward your opposite elbow. Be sure not to bend your neck and head forward. Raise your knee only slightly at first. As you get stronger, you can raise your knee a few inches on each rep. Breathe normally or exhale on each repetition. This exercise is advanced, so don't try to lift your knee too high too soon.

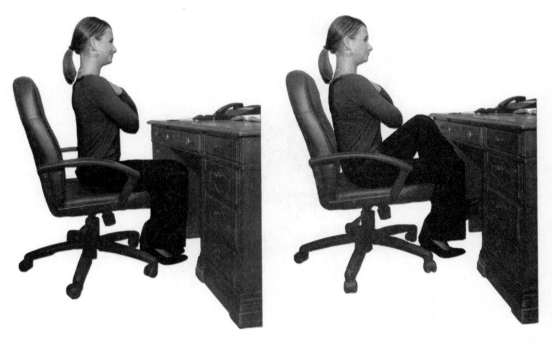

1. Fold your arms across your chest and sit up straight with your feet flat on the floor.

2. Raise your left knee toward your right elbow. Be sure to keep your back straight. Switch sides and repeat.

Using Your Desk—Side Abs

Using Your Desk—Side Abs trains the sides of your stomach. This exercise is very simple but it's not easy. Nobody should notice you doing this exercise if you are doing it correctly. Hold each repetition no longer than three seconds. Breathe normally or exhale on each repetition if you prefer. Keep your back straight and alternate sides so you do not strain the muscles in the tops of your thighs. Use your armrests for balance.

Although this exercise seems similar to Using Your Desk—Front Abs, it targets different muscle groups. When you raise both knees and press them against the desk, you are targeting your lower six-pack, rectus abdominis. When you raise one knee to contact your desk, your side abdominal oblique muscles are the prime movers.

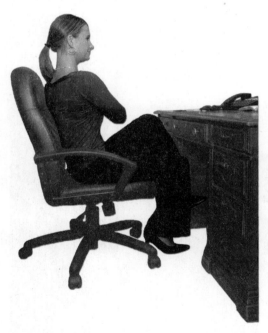

1. Sit on the front edge of your chair and lift your right knee so the upper-right thigh contacts your desk.

2. Switch legs and repeat.

Chair Exercise—Side Abs 2

The Chair Exercise—Side Abs 2 exercise tones the sides of your waist from a different angle. Keep your back straight and your neck relaxed. Your head should be aligned with your shoulders. Don't twist too far. Although you may use this move as a stretching exercise, flex your abs to make it a toning workout. At first, alternate sides rather than performing multiple repetitions on the same side. To increase the intensity of this exercise, perform multiple repetitions consecutively on the same side. Be sure to exhale on each repetition. To add a further challenge, let go of the armrest when you feel a maximal contraction of your abs and pause for one second.

GET IT RIGHT

Whiplash-type injuries may occur from doing stomach exercises too fast.

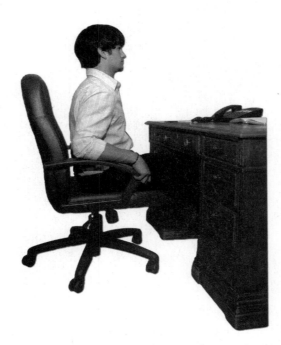

1. Grab the left armrest with your right hand. Twist to your left and flex the left side of your stomach for three seconds.

2. Grab the right armrest with your left hand. Twist to your right and flex the side of your stomach for three seconds.

Chair Exercise—Advanced Side Abs 2

Chair Exercise—Advanced Side Abs 2 trains the muscles on the sides of your stomach. Be careful not to lean your body too far to the side. Keep your back straight between reps. To increase the intensity of this exercise, place your fingers behind your head. Do not pull on your head with your hands. Exhale through each repetition. It is extremely important not to bend your neck; instead, tilt from your waist.

To add a further challenge, when you feel a maximal contraction of your abs, pause for a one-second count.

1. Cross your arms over your chest and keep your back straight, stomach in, and chest out.

2. Tilt your upper body to the right while lifting your right knee toward that elbow.

3. Tilt your upper body to the left while lifting your left knee toward that elbow. Don't try to bend too far.

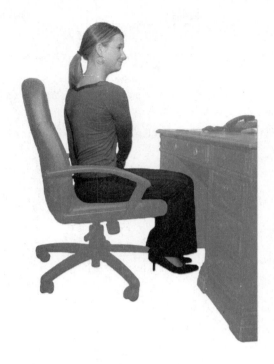

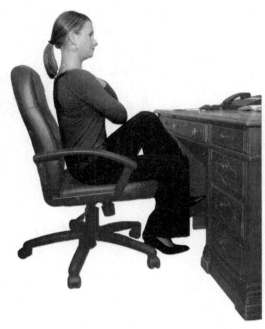

The Least You Need to Know

- Many seated ab exercises can be done without anyone else noticing you're doing them.
- To make seated ab exercises more challenging, add resistance or hold each position for a few seconds.
- A slight variation of an ab exercise can add difficulty or target different ab muscles.

Becoming Toned and Tight

13

In This Chapter

- Doing ab exercises at the gym
- Paying attention to your form
- Tightening your waistline

Home and office training is fine, but training your abs in the gym will get you to the next level. It's nice to be in the company of like-minded people. Some people go to the gym simply to be inspired by hard bodies they admire. Be careful, however, of the well-meaning wannabe bodybuilder attempting to share his latest ab-blasting workout. Take this book to the gym and compare his suggestions to our tried-and-true methods.

There is nothing like "feeling the burn" on that tenth rep. Maintain perfect form on every exercise. Move through a full range of motion, paying particular attention to keeping your neck relaxed. Depending on the exercise, your lower back should either be pressed to the floor or in its natural curve. Begin each exercise by using your lower-abdominal muscles to draw your navel toward your spine. Continue to flex these muscles through the duration of each repetition. If you cannot perform 10 repetitions with perfect form, decrease the amount of weight you are using. Breathe normally at first, but when the going gets tough, exhale on the exertion part of each repetition. When you can perform 10 repetitions with perfect form, it's time to add a couple pounds of resistance.

Seated Crunches with Resistance Bands

Seated Crunches with Resistance Bands trains the front of your stomach. The added resistance from the bands firms and tones your muscles. Anchor the exercise band securely. Concentrate on flexing your abs at the beginning of your rep. Keep tension on your abs throughout the duration of your set without resting in the up or down position. Move very slowly through each rep: three seconds down, three seconds up. Keep your elbows tucked into your body. Be careful not to pull with your arms. Sit with perfect posture between each rep. Round your back on each repetition. Curl your chest toward your legs. As your stomach muscles get stronger, add more resistance.

IN OTHER WORDS

Besides your six-pack, the muscles on the sides of your stomach (external and internal obliques) and your coughing muscle (transverse abdominis) are important for every move you make.

1. Begin in a seated position holding the handles of your resistance bands at neck level. The bands attach to the wall above head level.

2. Lean forward from your waist until you reach a 45-degree angle. As you exhale, keep your back straight and your chin off of your chest.

3. Return to your starting position and complete your repetitions.

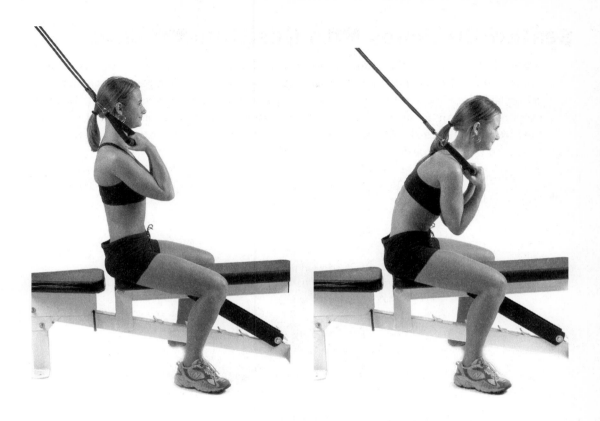

Roll Up

The Roll Up trains the muscles in the front of your stomach. This is a fun exercise you can do with your kids. It is relatively easy to do, so you may perform more than 10 reps if you wish. It's a great warm-up or cool-down exercise for your abs. Roll as slowly as you can; three seconds in both directions minimizes momentum. Be sure you are rolling on a mat or thick carpet. Keep your chin tucked to your chest and be careful not to roll too far in either direction.

Have fun with this one.

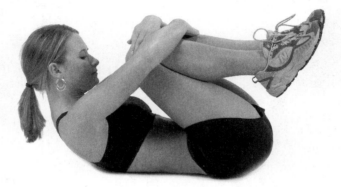

1. Lie on your back with your knees tucked into your chest.

2. Wrap your arms around your legs and begin rolling back and forth.

Butterfly Crunch

The Butterfly Crunch trains the muscles in the front of your stomach. Although this exercise looks kind of funny, it's awesome for your abs. You place the soles of your feet together to keep your upper-leg muscles from helping your abs out. Because your legs can't help, your abs are doing all of the work. Keep your back flat on the floor and begin each rep by contracting your stomach muscles. Curl your chest a couple inches toward your legs on each repetition.

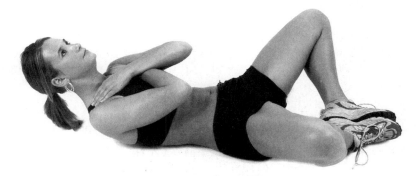

1. Lie on your back with your arms crossed over your chest.

2. Place the soles of your feet together as close to your body as possible with your knees bent.

3. Imagine you have an apple tucked between your chin and your chest and raise your shoulder blades a few inches off the floor.

4. Hold, then lower your back slowly to the floor.

BET YOU DIDN'T KNOW

If you miss a workout, no sweat. It is not one workout that matters, it is the weeks and months of training that make a difference.

Leg Raise

The Leg Raise tones the lower part of your stomach. Begin with your legs pointing straight up in the air with your knees slightly bent. Slowly lower your legs toward the floor. To prevent lower-back pain, be sure your lower back is flat to the floor. If you have never done this exercise before, bend your knees at 90 degrees. Find a range of movement that is comfortable, and be sure that your lower back does not come off the floor. If your lower back begins to arch, do not let your legs drop any farther. To prevent arching your back, you can tuck your hands underneath your rear end, and this will help keep your back flat.

Continue doing reps, beginning with your feet pointing toward the ceiling and then slowly lowering them. Three seconds up, three seconds down. Always stay in a range of motion where your back does not arch. Do these for 10 reps. Keep your neck relaxed through each rep. Breathe normally on this exercise. As you get stronger, you may extend your knees a little. Never fully extend your knees.

1. Lie on your back with your arms to your sides and your knees slightly bent.

2. Lift your legs toward the ceiling and lower them very slowly a few inches.

3. Return them to the starting position.

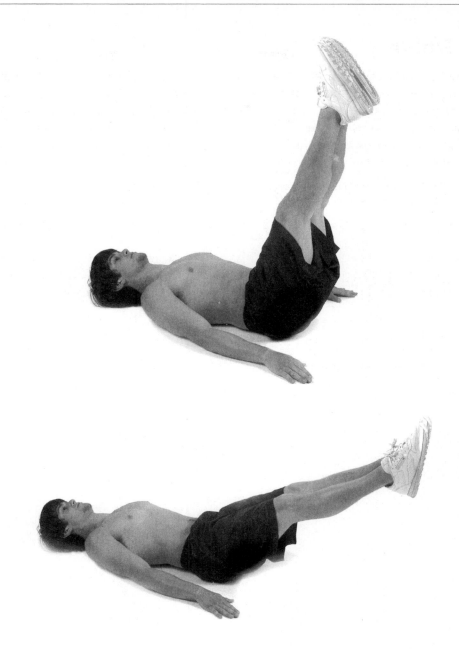

Leg Push

The Leg Push works the lower part of your stomach. Although it is a very small movement, be sure to maintain perfect form so that your lower-stomach muscles are working. If you cannot complete the three-second rep, begin with one-second reps. Add a second to each rep each week until you can perform 10 three-second reps. Be sure to breathe throughout each repetition and keep your back straight and neck relaxed.

1. Lie on your back with your arms to your sides and your feet pointed toward the ceiling.

2. Flex your lower-abdominal muscles so that your hips lift off the floor for three seconds.

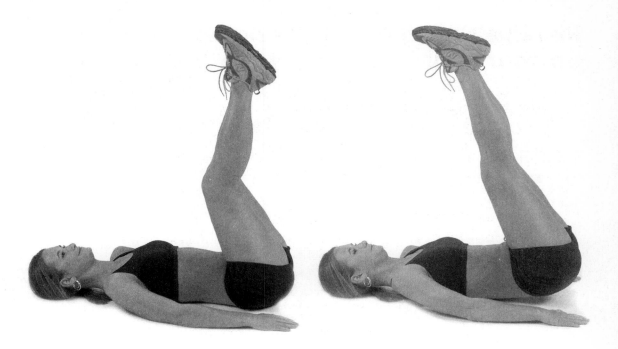

Reverse Crunches with Weights on Your Legs

Reverse Crunches with Weights on Your Legs tones the muscles of the lower pooch. Because gravity and stability are involved, you will be training other balancing muscles in your abs as well. Be sure the weights are secured to your legs. Don't try to lift too much too soon or you'll strain your upper-leg muscles. Because you are using weights instead of resistance bands, there will be a tendency for you to use momentum. Three seconds in both directions minimizes inertia.

GET IT RIGHT

Momentum is your worst enemy in the weight room. Move slowly to prevent injury and to be sure the correct muscles are working.

1. Lie on your back with your knees bent and ankle weights resting on the top of your ankles. Place your arms to your sides.

2. Lift your knees toward your chest, using your arms to balance until your hips leave the floor.

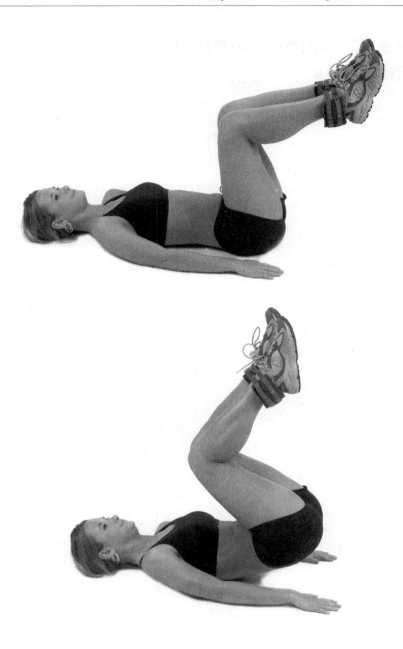

Reverse Crunches with Resistance Bands

Reverse Crunches with Resistance Bands train the lower part of your stomach underneath your navel (the pooch). Anchor the exercise band securely. Perform 10 repetitions with perfect form. Move three seconds in both directions. As your abs get stronger, add more resistance by doubling up on the band. As you add more resistance, work your way back up to 10 reps. Be sure to lift your hips off the floor at the end of each rep so that your legs are not doing the work that your abs are supposed to do.

1. Lie on your back with your knees bent and the resistance bands anchored to your ankles. Keep your arms to your sides.

2. Raise your knees toward your chest until your hips leave the floor.

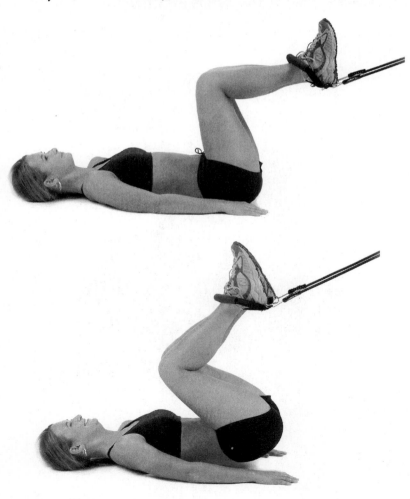

Twists with Resistance Bands

Twists with Resistance Bands train the sides of your stomach. This is a great exercise to firm and tone your entire waistline. These muscles are necessary for your daily activities, so the stronger the better. As your flexibility improves, you may twist a little further. Anchor the exercise band securely. Be sure to maintain perfect posture throughout the duration of each rep. Do not bend over from the waist. Move slowly and purposefully. Three seconds in both directions works great. Don't attempt to twist too far.

Perform 10 repetitions with perfect form. For a further challenge, as you get stronger, you may double the exercise band to add more resistance. Only add resistance when you can perform 10 reps without a break in your form.

1. Stand with your feet shoulder-width apart and your knees slightly bent. Hold the resistance band beside your waist.

2. Contract the sides of your stomach as you gently turn to the right. When you feel the contraction, stop and return to your original position.

3. Switch sides and repeat.

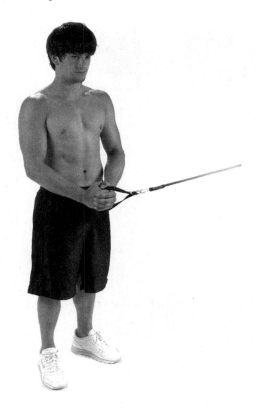

Side Planks

Side Planks train the sides of your stomach and lower-back muscles at the same time. Be sure to keep your body straight (don't sag) and hold for three seconds. If this exercise is too challenging from your feet, try it from the outside of your calf. If that is still too hard, do it from the side of your hip. Add 2 sets per week until you can perform 10 sets of three-second reps consecutively. At first, rest as long as you need to between sets. As you get stronger and develop more endurance, decrease the rest time between sets. Be sure to breathe normally during each repetition, or, if you prefer, you may exhale throughout the rep. You may decide to alternate right and left side planks to save time. As you get stronger, decrease the time between sets, and perform all of your planks on one side and then all of your planks on the other side.

1. Lie on your side bracing your body with your forearm and the outside edge of your shoe.

2. Lift your hip off of the floor and hold your body straight.

3. Switch sides and repeat.

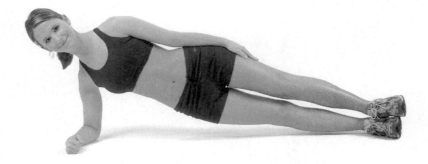

Front Plank

Front Plank trains all of your stomach muscles and your back as well. Be sure to keep your back straight and neck relaxed. Your back and neck will have a tendency to sag. Hold for three seconds. If you have a break in your form, stop the exercise immediately. Add 2 sets per week until you can perform 10 sets of three-second reps consecutively. At first, rest as long as you need to between sets. As you get stronger and develop more endurance, decrease the rest time between sets. Be sure to breathe normally during each repetition. If this exercise is too difficult, do it from your knees instead of your feet.

1. Start from your hands and knees and then slowly drop to your forearms and the balls of your feet. Keep your elbows in line with your shoulders. Some people prefer to clasp their hands together making a triangle, rather than having fingertips facing forward.

2. Contract your stomach and back muscles, but keep the rest of your body relaxed.

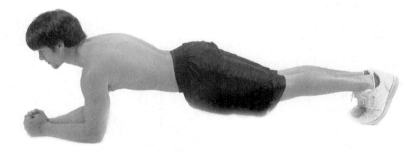

Shoulder Bridge

Shoulder Bridge trains your stomach and back muscles. Keep your feet hip-width apart. Your heels should be directly under your knees, your arms to your sides. Pull your navel toward your spine and, without arching your back, lift your hips toward the ceiling. Your body should form a straight, slanted line from your knees to your chest. Hold the bridge position for three seconds. Add 2 sets per week until you can perform 10 sets of three-second reps consecutively. Your neck and shoulders should be straight. Imagine you have an apple between your chin and your chest. At first, rest as long as you need to between sets. As you get stronger and develop more endurance, decrease the rest time between sets. Be sure to breathe normally during each repetition. If you prefer, you may exhale during the rep. Keep your hips elevated and level throughout the duration of the exercise.

YOUR PERSONAL TRAINER

For every exercise you do for your stomach, do two for your back. Fortunately, most of the exercises in this chapter train your back as well as your stomach so that you will maintain perfect balance and symmetry.

1. Lie down on your back with your knees bent and your arms to the sides. Press with your heels to lift yourself into the bridge or ramp position.

2. Keep your neck relaxed and your back straight.

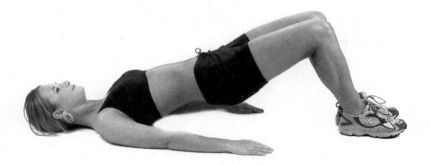

The Least You Need to Know

- Proper form is key, and when that can't be maintained any longer, stop the ab exercise.
- Work on holding each exercise for incrementally more seconds.
- Use weights and bands to add resistance.

Trim and Tone

In This Chapter

- Multi-tasking ab exercises
- Circuit training your abs
- Stretching your abs and back

Losing fat around your waist is easier than liposuction. You don't have to train until you're breathless or stay at a certain pace on the treadmill. You burn fat all day long. Little movements use energy and burn fat. Standing up and stretching, walking your dog, walking to the refrigerator—all incinerate fat. Figure out ways to add more movement into your day. The more you move, the better. In this chapter, you'll find ideas for working those abs during your everyday activities along with ab-isolation exercises to target your waistline.

One way to shed fat all day long is to flex your muscles. That's right, flex your abs whenever you think of it. Toned abs are rock-hard instead of flabby. Your abs will get firmer through conscious effort. If you keep your abs flexed they'll tend to stay firmer longer. Flexed abs use up more energy than relaxed abs. When your abs are flexed, there is more cross-bridging between your actin and myosin filaments. The small strands (actin) and large strands (myosin) in your muscle fibers are pulled together by cross-bridges. The more cross-bridging that's happening, the more chiseled and toned your abs are.

Commercial Crunches

A safe and effective way to train the front of your stomach while watching TV is the ubiquitous crunch. But to do a perfect crunch you have to maintain perfect form. The first part of the crunch is to flatten your lower back to the floor.

Put your hands on your abs to feel them work during the crunch. The crunch is a very small movement, and to others it might look like you're just goofing off and doing incomplete reps. But when summer comes, you'll be able to show them your sleek and chiseled six-pack.

You can get the most out of your stomach muscle exercises by bending your hips and knees to reduce the action of your hip flexors and to protect your lower back.

Placing your thighs at a right angle to your torso to begin with means that the hip flexors can't pull the torso any farther, so more of the work is done by your abs instead of your legs.

With your feet flat on the floor, press down and back with your heels. By pressing your heels into the floor you activate your hamstring muscles in the back of your leg. This keeps your hip flexor muscles from taking over for your abs.

BET YOU DIDN'T KNOW

It doesn't take 20 straight minutes of exercise to begin burning fat around your waist. Break your workouts into a few minutes each, scattered throughout your day.

Abs at Work

Chores are an ab workout, too. Find the most vigorous chores you can handle. Next time you rake leaves or sweep your driveway, focus on the toning effect on the sides of your stomach. When you lean to the side and pull, you are getting a great ab-isolation workout.

Next time you are doing the dishes, take notice that your abs are tight. Whether you are cleaning the counter or returning a milk jug to the refrigerator, you're training your abs.

YOUR PERSONAL TRAINER

Your body adapts to training, so change up your workout program occasionally.

Ab Circuits

Your ab-isolation training may be performed at home, in your office, or in the gym. Train your abs no more than every other day. Your ab-isolation exercises should take no longer than a few minutes.

How hard you train your abs is more important than how long. Go for "the burn" occasionally, but if your stomach muscles feel uncomfortable for a couple days, you went too far.

YOUR PERSONAL TRAINER

Start each movement slowly, as if you are in slow motion.

If you find yourself in a seated position and you only have a few minutes to train your abs, try this quick, 15-second ab-toning circuit. Circuit training is when you move from one exercise to the next as quickly as possible. Hold each position for three seconds.

Chair Circuit

Lean back until your stomach muscles contract, but don't touch the back of your chair. Then, without rest, bring your right foot off of the floor and your right knee toward your chest. Do the same with your left leg. For the final exercise, press your right forearm into your right armrest. Do the same with your left forearm.

In 15 seconds, you worked all of your ab muscles. If you have more time, simply do another circuit of the same routine. Three sets would be perfect.

Perform three ab-isolation exercises three times a week. Target each muscle with a specific exercise. Do three exercises per workout—one for your front abs, one for your side abs, and one that targets all of your stomach muscles simultaneously. Mix and match. Your abs love to be challenged from different angles and intensities. Use perfect form to maximize your progress and minimize soreness.

If you are extremely short on time, but you are at home or in the gym, put your ab-isolation exercises together into a floor circuit workout. This method of training keeps your heart rate up so that you tone your abs and lose belly fat simultaneously.

Floor Circuit

Lie on your back and do a set of 10 perfect crunches. Then, without any rest, do a set of 10 reverse crunches. Turn over on your stomach and hold a plank for 10 seconds. By now you might need a breather, so take a 30-second break and a sip of water. Then lie down on your side and hold a side plank for 10 seconds. Switch to your other side and hold a plank for 10 seconds.

And there you have it—a great ab-toning workout in less than 2 minutes (and that included your 30-second break).

Stretching Your Abs

General stretching is good for both your body and your brain. Blood flow is stimulated to increase your energy level. Through regular, active stretching, you will feel a greater sense of well-being, far greater vitality, and a calmer, more-relaxed attitude.

Stretching improves the elasticity of your abdominal muscles and ligaments surrounding your joints. It improves flexibility and helps to prevent injury and soreness. Stretching promotes muscular balance and relaxation and also decreases the resistance of your tissues.

Hold your stretch at least 10 seconds to fully relax the muscle. Breathe normally between each stretch; take deep breaths from your diaphragm and exhale into each stretch to nourish your muscles and aid in relaxation. Add 2 seconds a week until you work up to 30 seconds. Within months you may stretch to a slight level of tension but never approaching pain.

The following stretches engage your abdominals to maintain your balance and posture, in addition to stretching other areas of your body. Strong, flexible abdominals are essential for all of your active movements.

C-Stretch

The C-Stretch elongates your stomach muscles. Keep your neck aligned with your head and your shoulders down. Exhale into the deeper part of your stretch, but otherwise breathe normally. Be careful not to stretch too fast or too far. Stretch until you feel tension and then stop. If you are very flexible, you may extend the stretch by moving from your forearms to your hands. Press your hands into the floor and slowly extend your elbows until you feel tension. Always warm up before you stretch.

1. Lie on your stomach with your forearms under your shoulders and your palms on the floor.

2. Press your forearms into the floor as you raise your upper body, stretching from your waist. Hold for 30 seconds.

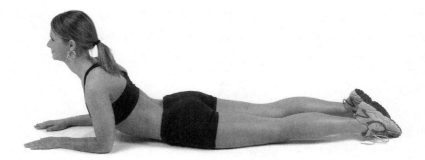

Upper-Thigh Stretch

The Upper-Thigh Stretch lengthens the muscles in the upper-front part of your leg called the hip flexors. Begin in a lunge position with your front leg bent at 90 degrees and your back leg straight. Keep your back straight and neck relaxed. Lean into your front leg. Be careful that your knee does not travel over your toe. Lean your upper body back slightly, tilting your pelvis forward. Breathe normally, but exhale into the deep part of the stretch.

YOUR PERSONAL TRAINER

Hold your stretch for 30 seconds to combat the myotatic response or stretch reflex. The stretch reflex is the rubber band–like recoil that you feel when you stretch a muscle too far too fast.

1. Stand with your left knee bent and your right leg straight behind you.

2. Tilt your pelvis forward and hold the stretch for 30 seconds.

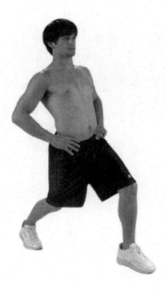

Lower-Back Flex

The Lower-Back Flex stretches out your lower back. If you do not bend down and bring your knees to your chest occasionally, you will lose the flexibility to perform this exercise. Many people from other countries possess outstanding flexibility because they squat in this position several hours a day. If this exercise puts too much pressure on your knees, you may do it from a side-lying position.

1. Squat on the floor with your knees to your chest.

2. Wrap your arms around your legs and bring your chin to your chest. Hold for 30 seconds.

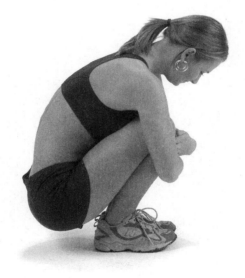

Lower-Back Arch

The Lower-Back Arch stretches all of the muscles in your back. You probably sit at your desk all day, sit at meals, and then sit for your morning and evening drive. The front of your body tightens up in this flexed position. To combat short, tight muscles, stretch them in the opposite direction. Keep your neck in line with your spine. Maintain a stable base by keeping your knees slightly bent. Perform this exercise several times a day. Do not lean back too far. Be sure to keep your head up to maintain your balance.

1. Stand with your feet shoulder-width apart and your arms out to the side.

2. Lean back with your chest high and hold for 30 seconds.

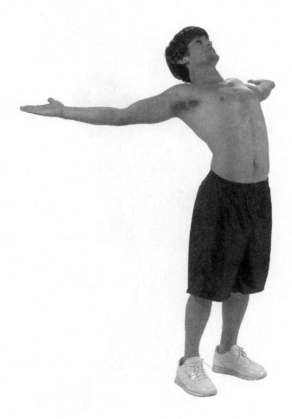

Back-of-Leg Stretch

The Back-of-Leg Stretch loosens up the muscles in the back of your upper leg. This exercise may be done while you are at work or if you are waiting in line. Perform this exercise several times a day to help keep your posture perfect. Stretching the backs of your legs also helps to prevent lower-back pain. Keep your back straight and your head up. Maintain a slight arch in your lower back with your hips back. Place both hands on the middle thigh of your supporting right leg.

1. Stand with your feet shoulder-width apart and your weight on your right leg. Keep your right knee bent.

2. Extend your left knee, hinge at the hip, and feel a stretch in the back of your left leg. Hold this stretch for 30 seconds.

3. Switch sides and repeat.

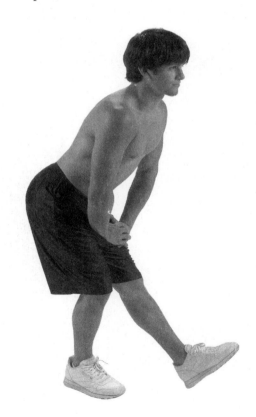

The Least You Need to Know

- Your abs are always working when you're active.
- Strong, flexible abs are necessary for good balance and posture.
- Be consistent doing ab-isolation exercises to see results.
- Ab muscles are engaged during stretching of different body parts.

Buns and Thighs

This part explores exercises you can do at home, the gym, and the office to tone and tighten the muscles in your legs, thighs, and butt—including hamstrings, glutes, and hips. You'll also learn stretches for buns, thighs, and legs to help maximize your workouts.

Buns and Thighs Made Simple

In This Chapter

- The "sweep" of the thigh
- The way to remember your hamstrings
- The way to understand butt muscles
- The connection of hips and inner thighs

The perfect body is an "X" shape. The top of the X are your shoulders and upper back, narrowing into your waist and hips. The bottom of the X are long legs with upper thighs that appear to connect directly to the waist. The legs are the most important part to develop. When trained correctly, they make your waist look smaller and complete the X shape.

Everyone loves a nice pair of legs. What you do with them, however, will greatly affect how they look. The hips, butt, and thighs are the problem areas, where women accumulate most of their cellulite. Unfortunately for women, nature has designated fat cells in the lower body to serve as energy storage for pregnancy and lactation.

Men generally store most of their fat in their bellies. They try to build up their chests and arms to compensate. But nothing looks more ridiculous than a guy whose arms are bigger than his legs.

Many women fear they will get bulky legs if they lift weights, but you won't get "bulky" if you train correctly. You may actually lose size by lifting weights because you become more compact. When training, it's important not only to know where your muscles are, but also what they do so you can sculpt them accordingly. Following is a brief overview of the lower-body muscles.

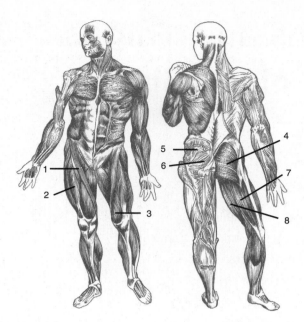

1. Adductors (inner upper thighs)
2. Rectus femoris (middle thigh)
3. Vastus medialis (inner lower thigh)
4. Gluteus maximus (backside)

5. Gluteus minimus (side of butt—inner)
6. Gluteus medius (side of butt—outer)
7. Biceps femoris (middle hamstrings)
8. Semitendinosus (inner hamstrings)

The muscle groups in the buns and thighs.

Thighs

Female fashion models are tall with very long legs. Believe it or not, some people are born this way! Others, unfortunately, are somewhere on the continuum between "model" legs and thick, short, stubby legs. If you weren't born with the genetics of a model, you can get closer to the long-legged look by weight training.

If you have decent leg development in proportion to the rest of your body, you'll look sexy. And although your thigh muscles require intense workouts to see results, your goal is to keep your whole body in proportion.

Train your entire thigh from top to bottom. Check out people at the beach and you will see "carrot thighs"—big on top and in the middle, but no development in the lower thigh. A well-shaped thigh should be nearly as wide at the bottom part as at the mid part. Carrot-shaped legs can throw off your symmetry. A good thigh sweep will offset a thick waist. In bodybuilding, the "sweep" refers to the symmetrical development of the outer thigh muscle (*vastus lateralis*) and the lower part of the hourglass shape—the larger the chest and back and the larger the hips and thigh sweep, the smaller the waistline appears.

The *quads* are the front part of the thighs, and as the name implies, consist of four muscles. The *rectus femoris*, the large muscle in the center of the thigh, crosses both the knee and hip. It connects from your pelvis to below the kneecap. This muscle can help you bend your hip or straighten your knee.

The *vastus lateralis* is your very visible outer thigh muscle. This muscle provides the "sweep"—the lower part of the "X" that creates the illusion that your legs attach directly to your waist. When you have well-defined legs, there is a perceptible separation between this muscle and the hamstrings muscle in the back of your legs. A good thigh sweep will offset a thick waist.

Your *vastus medialis* is on the inside of your thigh. It creates that "teardrop" appearance just above the knee. Keep this muscle strong to prevent knee problems and to balance out your entire set of thigh muscles.

The *vastus intermedius*, underneath the rectus femoris, runs from the top of the thighbone to the knee and works to straighten the knee. Place your right hand on your right thigh. Extend your right foot out in front. You can feel the vastus intermedius and your other thigh muscles flexing. These large muscles can be compared to the muscle on the back of your upper arm. That is, by flexing, they straighten the leg.

Different foot positioning during leg exercises targets different areas of the thighs. For greater overall development of the front thigh, keep your toes pointed forward and have your feet just outside your shoulders. Pointing the toes out with a wide stance targets the glutes as well. To firm your inner thighs, point your toes out but keep your feet closer. For outer thigh development (the sweep), keep your legs close and toes pointed straight ahead.

Heavy squats and partial range of motion leg presses develop the upper thigh, hips, and butt. The teardrop-shaped lower-thigh muscle can be developed with a narrower stance. The front squat shapes the upper thigh because it targets your rectus femoris, which goes all the way up to your hips. When this muscle is developed, it makes your legs appear longer.

GET IT RIGHT

Balancing the size and strength between your thighs and hamstrings not only keeps your legs looking great, but it protects the stability of your knees.

Hamstrings

In gyms you may notice lines of people waiting at the bench press while the hamstring machine sits idle. Many males who work out to build size are concerned with getting their chests huge and biceps bulging, and often place too much emphasis on their arm workouts while neglecting to do anything for their hamstrings. What they may not realize is that if they train their legs, the muscles of the upper body are stimulated, too.

To get defined arms, you work your biceps. Your hamstrings are considered your leg biceps. A thick, rounded set of hamstrings are muscles that stand out.

Women have a different reason to train their hamstrings—cellulite. Every woman has cellulite. Cellulite is simply fat, water, and toxins under the tissue beneath the skin, causing that "cottage cheese" appearance.

Whether you want to build muscle, lose fat, or incinerate cellulite, your hamstrings workout is a huge part of the solution. Legs, as a whole, are neglected, but the hamstrings are the forlorn stepchildren. The hamstrings lie along the length of your rear thigh. They connect near the butt and the back of the knee. Leg flexing or bending uses the hamstrings muscles. They act in the same manner as the front of your arm (ergo leg biceps).

The three muscles of your hamstrings are the *biceps femoris*, *semitendinosus*, and *semimembranosus*.

The bicep femoris (leg biceps) is the outer sweep of the hamstring. When you turn sideways, this is the muscle that gives your leg that full, sexy look. It has two heads; the long head crosses the knee and the hip, and the short one only crosses the knee. These muscles curl the lower leg up toward your butt, and work with your butt muscles to straighten your hip.

As much as you may hate training your hamstrings, it is the most impressive part of your upper leg. Nothing looks better than seeing a firm, rounded group of hamstrings muscles. To improve the lines and symmetry in your hamstrings, train with enough weight that the tenth repetition is a challenge. Your hamstrings are mostly fast-twitch muscle fibers.

IN OTHER WORDS

Fast-twitch, type IIB fibers are white, powerful, and larger than the slow-twitch, type I, red endurance fibers.

If you want your hamstrings to be round and full, train them by doing leg curls. The secret to filling out your hamstring muscle is to keep your ankles relaxed. If you flex your ankle, you use your calf muscle in your lower leg to do the work that the hamstrings are supposed to do.

Train your hamstrings at different angles and intensities to get full development. You can vary your toe position when doing exercises to target different areas of your hamstrings. When you add density to your hamstrings, you create a perfect balance with your thighs.

Buns

If you were born with a round bottom, you lucked out. If you don't have buns of steel, you are not alone. Stand up and take a good look at your butt. You probably think that it is too small, too saggy, too flabby, or too big. Maintaining your shapely buns is a fight against gravity. Owning a great set of buns is hot, but cellulite is not. Imagine cellulite on the outside of your butt as a wrinkled-up, old balloon. Your butt muscles are the air in the balloon. If you blow up the rubber balloon by firming up your muscles, the wrinkles go away and the rubber on the balloon gets thinner.

YOUR PERSONAL TRAINER

Firm those buns all day long. Whenever you are about to sit, stand, stoop, or bend down, lead with your buns and keep your back straight.

Although aerobic exercise burns calories, lower-body resistance training is a quick way to tone muscle and help reduce cellulite. By firming the butt muscles below the fat, the cellulite on top of the muscle thins out.

The *gluteus maximus* (butt muscle) is the largest and most superficial of the three buttocks muscles that form the gluteal complex, or glutes. So that's where most of your firming will take place. The glutes originate on the back of your pelvis and attach to the rear thighbone. The glutes are the muscles responsible for moving your legs backward and outward. They are the most powerful muscles in the body. You use your gluteals whenever you step, sit, or stand. While standing, place your right hand on your right bun and raise your right leg backward a couple inches off of the floor. Feel your glutes flex? This is the muscle that gives your butt that lifted look.

Straightening your legs from a bent-knee position requires you to straighten your hip. This is a major function of your glutes. Stand up from your chair and you will feel your glutes tighten. If you want to really activate your glutes, press through your heels when you stand up. You just performed the up phase of a squat called hip extension.

Unlike muscles such as the thigh, the glutes are nearly impossible to train by themselves. When you train your thighs or hamstrings, your glutes usually help. Because butt firming and toning is a side effect of training your legs, you may not have to give them a second thought.

Even without butt-specific training, you may already have firm, tight buns from everything else you do. But if you don't have the firm butt you desire, small adjustments in your leg workouts can maximize your gluteus maximus.

BET YOU DIDN'T KNOW

Lifting weights tightens, trims, and firms muscle, with no worries of developing a big butt. If you train properly, you can actually lose inches. Women are generally stronger in their lower body than in their upper body, so they should make sure to train with lower weights/high reps. This will keep them from building too much muscle, and keep their body in proportion.

For instance, you can maximize gluteal stimulation during the squat by adopting a wider stance. From a wide stance, you increase hip extension and decrease knee extension, so the emphasis shifts somewhat from your thighs to your glutes.

Outer Hips

Some people gain cellulite in their lower body while others gain fat around their midsection. You have probably heard about pear-shaped and apple-shaped body types, but there is more to your anatomical structure than just fat deposits.

If you have trouble with your saddlebags, flat fanny, thunder-thighs, or bubble buns, change your silhouette by training your gluteal muscles layer by layer. Although you cannot lose your saddlebags on the outer hip by working them, if you tone the muscle underneath the fat, there is an appearance of spot reduction. This is because the overlying fat is stretched over a greater surface due to your increased muscle tone. Your outer hips appear thinner, although the total amount of fat stays the same.

Place your right hand on the side of your right hip. Raise your right leg out to the right side. The muscle that you feel flexing is your hip abductor. It is part of the upper hip. This is the muscle that firms your saddlebag area. It is also called the *gluteus medius.*

The gluteus medius lies under the gluteus maximus and adds to the roundness of your butt. This muscle connects from the upper pelvis to the upper edge of your thighbone. The *gluteus minimus* is a smaller muscle that lies underneath the gluteus medius.

These muscles are easy to tone up using isolation exercises. But their most important function is to balance your movement during lunges and squats. These balancing muscles help with other glute-toning activities that you do outside of the gym, such as walking and hiking.

Inner Thighs

If you were asked to demonstrate your muscularity, you would probably flex your upper arm rather than your inner thigh. Flabby inner thighs are common. Fat and muscle are two separate entities and there is no magic formula to change fat into muscle.

You can't change how your muscles attach, your bone structure, or other hereditary factors, but you can certainly change the overall shape and definition of your inner thighs and improve your symmetry. You can sculpt your inner thigh muscles into a work of art.

Your inner thigh muscles are found deep in the inner groin and along the inner thigh. They are noticeably larger than the hamstrings and are almost as big as the quads. Your inner thigh muscles are easy to feel with your own hands. Place the palm of your hand on the inside of your thigh. Press your knees together and you will feel the large tendon become firm as the muscles pull taut. Trace the firm shape of the flexed muscles almost all the way down to your knee.

The five muscles that make up the inner thighs are collectively called the *hip adductors,* named after the movement they perform, which is bringing the legs toward and across the midline of the body. Individually, these muscles are the *adductors magnus, longus,* and *brevis;* the *gracilis;* and the *pectineus.* The latter two are also hip flexor muscles.

All five muscles attach from the pubis bone and ischial tuberosities (sit bones) and connect to the thighbone. Two of the adductors, the pectineus and the adductor brevis, are quite short and are connected to the back of the upper thighbone. The adductor longus and adductor magnus are longer and larger, and connect at the back of the lower thighbone. The longest adductor, the gracilis, inserts below the knee, on the inner upper shinbone. Together, all five of these muscles pull the thighs together. Several of them also have good leverage to flex the hip, pulling the thigh and torso toward each other.

The inner thigh muscles help you to keep your balance and are used for walking, standing, or climbing. The other actions of the inner thigh muscles are quite complicated. Depending on the position of the leg, they may also help rotate the thighbone internally or externally in the hip socket, or help straighten the hip.

The Least You Need to Know

- A well-shaped thigh is nearly as wide at the bottom part as it is in the middle part.
- Working the hamstrings is essential for toned and defined legs, yet they are often neglected in workouts.
- Lower-body resistance training is a quick way to tone muscle and help reduce cellulite.
- Outer hips can be toned using isolation exercises.

Buns and Thighs at Home

In This Chapter

- Making the most of household chores
- Discovering the power of the squat and lunge
- Toning your buns on the floor

Your buns and thighs are the foundation of your body. And there's no better place to build a foundation than in your living room. Bun and thigh training at home is an adventure in creative exercise. Perform traditional squats and lunges, but firm your buns and thighs by also climbing stairs and doing chores. Tone your buns and thighs throughout the day or designate a specific time for your training. If you choose the latter, let the answering machine take your calls, have water available, lock the doors, and begin.

On all home bun and thigh exercises, keep your back straight and stomach in. Imagine a piece of dental floss tied around your waist while performing every exercise. Use your lower abs to flex your navel in toward your spine. Exhale on the exertion of each rep. Keep your neck relaxed and maintain your concentration throughout each repetition.

Lift a Pencil Off the Floor

Lifting a Pencil Off the Floor doesn't seem like much of an exercise, but it is the perfect movement to train your buns and thighs. In fact, consider *any* lifting movement as a buns and thigh toner.

The hard part about doing this exercise is to maintain perfect form when it's a lot easier to cheat by bending from your waist. Although the pencil is not very heavy, use perfect form through the movement. When most people pick up a pencil from the floor, they bend and twist their spine—not very healthy for your back. Keep your head up, chest out, and stomach in. Bend your knees and lead with your hips.

IN OTHER WORDS

Your gluteus maximus (glutes) refers to your buns, while your quadriceps (quads) are the four large muscles on the front of your thigh.

1. Move in close to the pencil and spread your feet at least shoulder-width apart.

2. Squat as if into a chair and pick up the pencil.

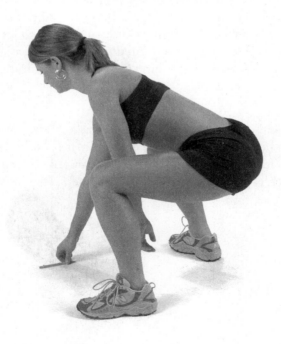

Free Squat

The Free Squat is the single best exercise to isolate your buns, thighs, hamstrings, and outer and inner thighs. Squat as if you were sitting back into a chair. Keep your upper body lifted with your shoulders back and head up. Always lead with your hips. There is no need to squat past a position where your thighs are parallel to the floor. Be sure that your knees do not travel over your toes and keep your knees in line with your toes. Don't worry how far you descend. That will depend on your limb and torso length and your flexibility. If you begin to lean forward, or your knees draw inward, return to your starting position.

1. Place your hands on your hips and spread your feet shoulder-width apart. Keep your chest out and eyes looking over the horizon.

2. Press through your heels and sit back as if into a chair until your thighs are parallel to the floor. If your knees begin to travel over your toes or you lose your form, stop immediately and slowly move back into your original position.

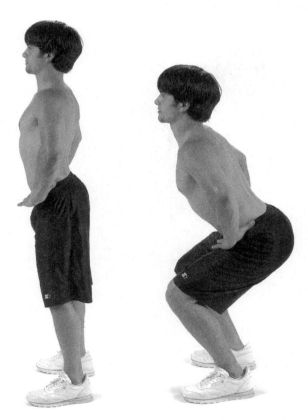

Lunge

The Lunge firms your thighs, buns, hamstrings, and inner and outer thighs. The Lunge is an athletic move that requires you to use balancing muscles. Pull your shoulders back and toward each other. Stay perfectly aligned so the exercise targets your legs and buns instead of your lower back. Keep your chest and head up. Resist the temptation to look down at your feet. Imagine an apple tucked between your chin and your chest.

Focus on your front leg as the workhorse for this exercise. Your back leg is there for balance. Don't go down too far if you have any problems with your knees or ankles. Maintain a 90-degree angle with your ankle, knee, and hip. Be sure your knees do not travel beyond your toes. At first, you may just bend down to a 45-degree angle with your knees. As you get stronger, you may descend to a position of 90 degrees.

YOUR PERSONAL TRAINER

Do squats and lunges whenever you can because they are the best exercises to firm all of your bun and thigh muscles, including your inner and outer thighs.

1. Step forward with your right foot as if you were straddling a railroad track. Keep your chest out and eyes forward.

2. Press through the heel of your front foot. Bend both knees to a 90-degree angle. Be sure your knees do not travel beyond your toes. Switch legs and repeat.

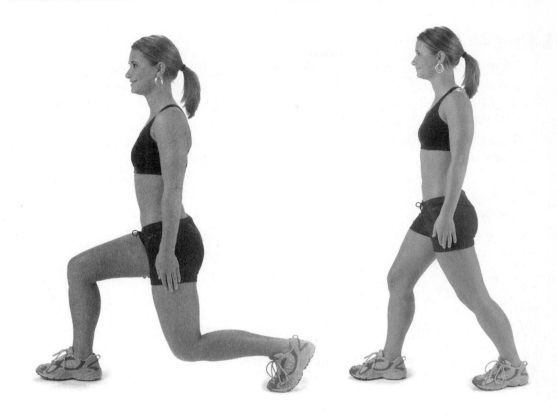

Chores

Chores such as loading the dishwasher tone your thighs, buns, hamstrings, and inner and outer thighs if you bend down with perfect form. Simulate squats and lunges on every lifting or lowering movement. You can get a great workout in the kitchen. Keep your center of gravity over your hips.

Whether you are putting away dishes or lifting a watermelon from the bottom of the refrigerator, move slowly and purposefully, as if you were in slow motion. Concentrate on the muscles that are working. Be careful not to reach or rush through the movements. Treat these movements with the same care that you would any other exercise.

1. Get as close as possible to the dishwasher. Bend from your hips, knees, and ankles.

2. Instead of reaching, step into your lift.

GET IT RIGHT

Train your thighs and hamstrings equally to prevent a muscle imbalance, which could cause a knee injury.

Climbing Stairs

Climbing Stairs tones your thighs, buns, hamstrings, and inner and outer thighs. If you have stairs in your home, you don't need a stair-climbing machine. Focus on toning your thighs by staying on the balls of your feet. To firm your buns, press through your heels on each step. Use the handrails for balance only. Do not pull on the handrails.

For advanced stepping, walk upstairs backward. Use the handrail for balance until you master this technique. Keep your form perfect, just as you would for any other exercise. Move in slow motion. As a change of pace you may side-step up and down the stairs. Train the same muscles at different angles.

1. Use the handrail for balance, step through your heel, and keep your head and chest up.

Back Wall Press

The Back Wall Press firms your buns and hamstrings. (This was a punishment exercise in elementary school!) While your hips are against the wall, you have the choice to target-tone your thighs or your hamstrings. For thigh work, center your weight on the balls of your feet. To burn your buns, shift your weight to your heels.

To train both your thighs and buns, shift your weight back and forth. Keep your eyes forward, your shoulders down, and your upper body relaxed. Your back should retain its natural curve. If your knees bother you on this exercise, bend your knees at 45 degrees instead of 90 degrees.

1. Stand with your back against a wall and slowly lower your hips until your knees are bent at 90 degrees.

2. Press through your heels in order to target your buns.

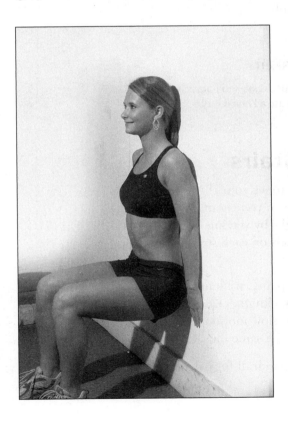

Lying on Your Back Buns Blaster

The Lying on Your Back Buns Blaster targets your buns and hamstrings. Do not arch your back or lift your hips too high. This is a great exercise to do when you don't want people to know you're working out; it's a very subtle movement.

On each rep, draw your navel into your spine and hold the contraction throughout the duration of the exercise. This exercise may be accomplished with both legs or one leg at a time. You can do this while watching television or reading in bed.

IN OTHER WORDS

Resistance training is the best tool to reshape your buns and thighs. Cardio is second best.

1. Lie on your back with your legs together and your knees slightly bent.

2. Press your heels into the floor and hold for three seconds.

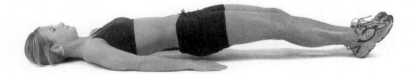

Lying on Your Stomach Buns Blaster

Lying on Your Stomach Buns Blaster trains your buns and hamstrings. Begin this exercise by drawing your navel into your spine. Flex your buns as you begin to lift your legs off of the floor. Lift them no higher than an inch off of the floor. Be careful not to hold your breath on this exercise. Instead, exhale through pursed lips throughout each rep.

If this exercise feels too difficult, do one leg at a time and alternate legs. After you have mastered this exercise and are ready for a challenge, add some weight to your ankles.

1. Lie on your stomach with your arms to your sides. Turn your head to one side.

2. Lift your legs and be sure you are hinging from your hip. Hold for three seconds.

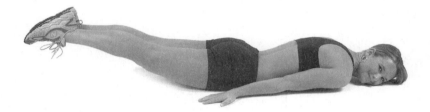

Side Wall Press

The Side Wall Press firms the outside of your hips (saddlebags). If this muscle doesn't get enough stimulation, it loses its tone. A toned hip muscle adds shape to your bottom. As you get stronger, you may press harder into the wall. Pressing harder is like adding weight on a weight machine. At first, hold on to the wall with your hand for balance.

Begin each exercise by drawing your navel into your spine. Flex the side of your hip to begin the movement. Exhale through the duration of each rep.

After you have mastered the exercise, allow your supporting leg to provide stability and let go with your hand. When you can do this exercise without holding on, you are training the outside of the hips of both legs simultaneously. Pay attention to your posture and keep your upper body relaxed.

1. Stand straight, with your left foot 3 inches away from a wall. Your left side is facing the wall.

2. Press the edge of your left foot into the wall and hold for three seconds. Switch legs and repeat.

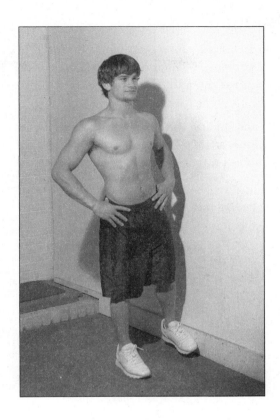

Back Heel Press

The Back Heel Press firms your buns and hamstrings. Begin each exercise by drawing your navel into your spine. Similar to the Side Wall Press, gradually increase how hard you press against the wall. Keep your back straight and exhale through the duration of each rep.

For this exercise, do not hold on to the wall for balance. Allow your supporting leg to stabilize your movement. This gives your supporting leg a workout, too. Maintain perfect posture and focus on firming your buns.

1. Stand 3 inches in front of a wall and extend your right leg back until the back edge of your heel makes contact.

2. Press and hold for three seconds. Switch legs and repeat.

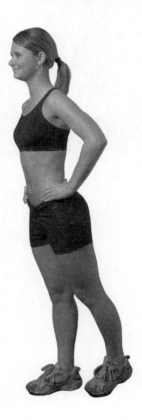

The Least You Need to Know

- The Free Squat and the Lunge work all around the bun and thigh muscles.
- Everyday actions like doing chores and climbing stairs work the buns and thighs, so pay attention to your form when you're doing them to maximize the benefit.
- Maintain a straight back during lower-body exercises.

Buns and Thighs at the Office

In This Chapter

- Combating saddlebags while you work
- Finding that small movements yield big results
- Toning and firming under the desk

Sitting all day long is the worst thing you can do if you want to have great buns and thighs. Wouldn't it be great if you could firm your buns and thighs in your office chair while you're reading or typing?

Well, you can, and it's easy! You can even do these simple exercises while on the phone or during a live interview. All of the movements are subtle, but the toning and shaping effects are amazing.

Maintain perfect posture on every exercise. Be sure to breathe normally while you flex your target muscle. Hold each squeeze for three seconds. Perform 10 reps of each exercise. Keep your upper body relaxed. At first, while you're in the learning stage, concentrate fully on your form. After a few months you will be able to firm and tone while you multitask on your computer or conduct an interview.

Heel Press

The Heel Press firms your thighs, buns, and hamstrings. There's no learning curve on this great start-up exercise. Your office mates will have no idea you're toning your lower body. At first, press lightly into the floor. As you get stronger, challenge yourself to press harder. Breathe normally or exhale into each rep. Flex your lower abs into your spine to get even better results. Eventually you will feel as if you might be able to rise up out of the chair without using your armrests.

Keep your back straight and your head up. Wear flat shoes or kick them off. High heels won't work very well for this exercise. To spice things up, isolate each leg by performing alternating heel presses.

1. Bend your knees at 90 degrees and keep your feet flat on the floor.

2. Press your heels into the floor.

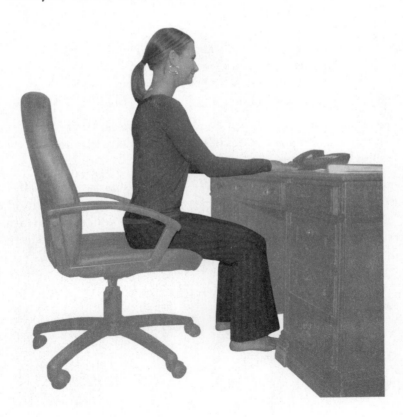

Outer Thigh Press

The Outer Thigh Press firms the sides of your hips (saddlebags) and buns. It's amazing how much you can firm and tone these muscles in the privacy of your office. You can also do this exercise while you're in a meeting or on the phone. After you practice for a couple weeks, your effort will be undetectable to others.

You can breathe normally or exhale into each rep. Flex your lower abs into your spine to get even better results. As you get stronger and are looking for a further challenge, press harder. Do not hunch over. Use your armrests to brace your effort if necessary. As a change of pace, alternate legs.

1. Sit at the front of your chair with your knees bent at 90 degrees and your feet together.

2. Place your hands on the outside of your knees and press the outside of your knees against your hands.

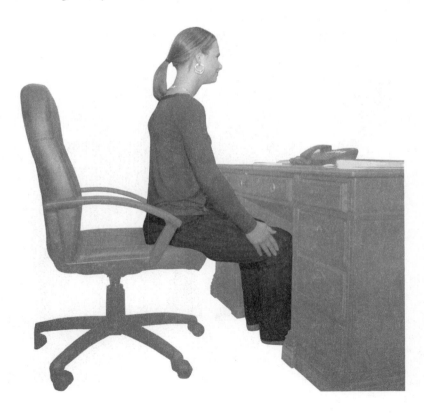

Figure-4 Press

The Figure-4 Press tones your outer thighs and buns. If someone saw you in this position, it would just look like you were relaxing or in deep thought. Little do they know you're spot-toning your hips and saddlebags!

Breathe normally or exhale into each rep. Flex your lower abs into your spine to get even better results. At first, use your arms to brace yourself if necessary. Adjust your ankle on your thigh to change the angle of the exercise. This recruits muscles at different angles to further your progress. At first, alternate legs after each rep. After a month of doing the exercise at least twice a week, perform all 10 reps on one side, then all 10 reps on the other side. Take as much rest as you need between reps.

1. Sit in a Figure-4 position with your right ankle resting on your left knee.

2. Press your ankle into your thigh. Repeat with your other leg.

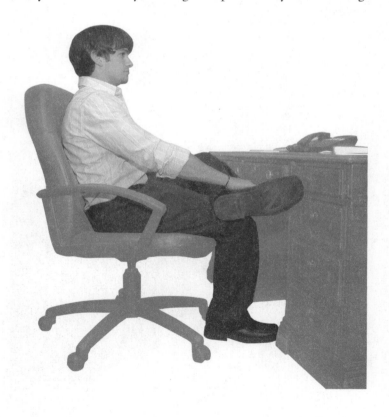

Cross Ankle

The Cross Ankle firms your outer thighs and buns. This is another great exercise that is imperceptible to others. Don't squeeze too tight at first. Breathe normally or exhale into each rep. Flex your lower abs into your spine to get even better results.

As you become stronger, squeeze harder. Do not lean forward or back on this exercise. At first, alternate legs after each rep. After a month of doing this exercise at least twice a week, perform all 10 reps on one side, then all 10 reps on the other side. Take as much rest as you need between reps.

1. Cross your right ankle over your left ankle with your knees together.

2. Press the outside edges of your feet together.

3. Cross your left ankle over your right ankle and repeat.

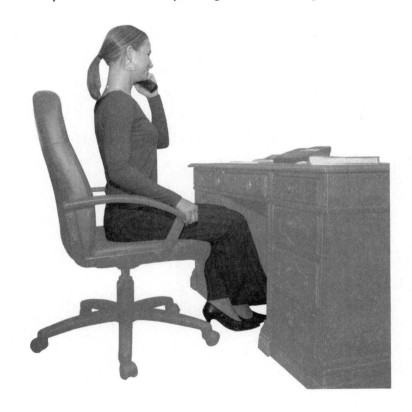

T-Press

The T-Press is a firming exercise for your inner thighs and hamstrings. In this exercise, both legs are working, so be sure to maintain perfect form and posture. Because both feet are resisting each other, there is a toning effect for both legs.

YOUR PERSONAL TRAINER

When performing your bun and thigh exercises, keep equal pressure on both legs to maintain proper symmetry and a shapely, balanced look.

At first, alternate legs between reps. After a month of doing this exercise at least twice a week, perform all 10 reps on one side, then all 10 reps on the other side. Take as much rest as you need between reps. Breathe normally or exhale into each rep. Flex your lower abs into your spine to get even better results.

1. Sit with your left foot pointed straight ahead and your left knee bent at 90 degrees.

2. Place the back heel of your right foot into the inside middle of your left foot. Your right foot should be pointed to the right and your right knee is slightly bent.

3. Press the back of your right heel into the middle of your left foot.

4. Switch legs and repeat.

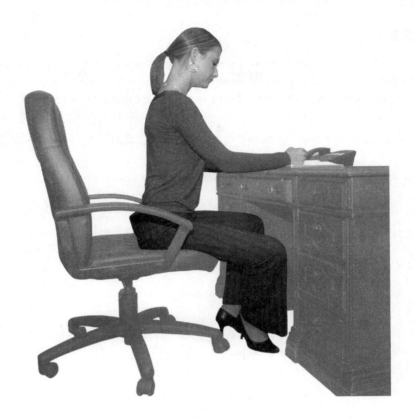

BET YOU DIDN'T KNOW

Fixing flabby inner thighs is as much a function of a proper diet as firming the muscle underneath the fat with toning exercises.

V-Press

The V-Press shapes your buns and inner thighs. At first, simply concentrate on pressing your heels together with your toes pointed outward. As you become more advanced, you may benefit your pelvic floor muscles while you perform this exercise by doing a Kegel. A Kegel is when you squeeze the muscles that you would use to stop urinating. To receive even greater benefit on this exercise, squeeze your bun cheeks together.

Breathe normally or exhale into each rep. Maintain perfect posture.

1. Sit with your heels together and your toes pointed slightly outward.

2. Press the inside of your heels together.

3. At the same time, press your heels into the floor.

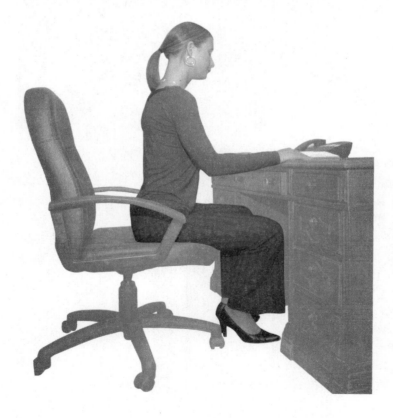

Bow-Legged

The Bow-Legged firms your inner thighs and buns. Do not slouch on this exercise. Be careful not to press too hard at first. Your inner thigh muscles are probably not used to this type of a workout. You may breathe normally or exhale into each rep.

Flex your lower abs into your spine to get even better results. Press lightly at first, and then as you get stronger you may press harder. Apply equal pressure with both legs.

1. Sit with the soles of your feet together and your knees bowed out.

2. Press the soles of your feet together.

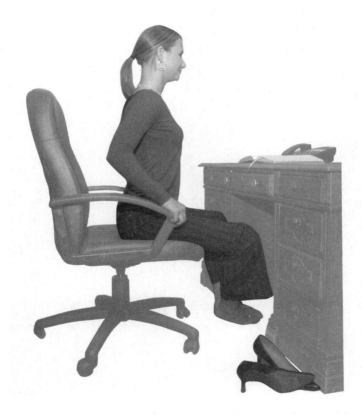

 GET IT RIGHT

Between sets of leg exercises, stand up and move around occasionally to get the kinks out and to speed the circulation in your lower body.

Inner Knee Press

The Inner Knee Press tones your inner thighs. No one will know that you are performing this exercise. Press your knees together until you feel tension. Breathe normally or exhale into each rep. Flex your lower abs into your spine to get even better results. As you get stronger, squeeze harder. Use your armrests for balance if necessary.

Maintain perfect posture throughout the duration of this exercise.

1. Sit with your feet and knees together.

2. Press your knees together.

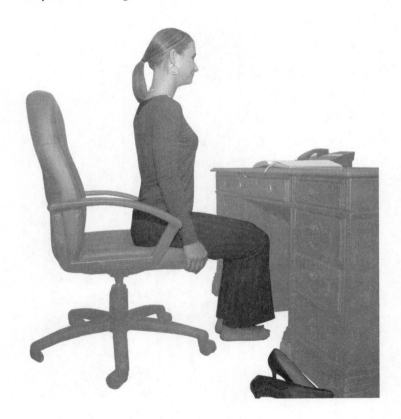

The Least You Need to Know

- Focus on proper form to make the most of each exercise.
- Increase the length of squeezing time to add challenge.
- Buns and thighs suffer with a desk job, but they don't have to with these exercises.

Buns and Thighs at the Gym

In This Chapter

- Toning exercises using benches, bars, and weights
- Using proper form and slow movement
- Tightening your butt and thighs

Don't be afraid of the gym. If you're concerned that you're the only one with sagging buns or flabby thighs, look around. Most people in the gym are just like you, trying to get to that next level: toned and tight. The most important thing is walking through the doors to make the commitment for your training program. Intimidation should not be a factor—most people are too absorbed in themselves and their own workout to pay attention to you!

Motivated gym-goers can inspire you when you would rather sit on the couch. Gyms are like social clubs—a place to meet new people—and many offer personal training and aerobics classes. If your gym is part of a chain, you can use their facilities in different cities. Gym machines have built-in safety features so that when you can no longer press a weight, you just set it down. Machines remove balance as a factor and ensure correct movements to isolate your buns and thighs. Changing the resistance on a machine is as easy as changing the pin.

Always maintain perfect posture. Keep your back straight, stomach in, chest out, and eyes forward. You will notice as many people doing exercises incorrectly as those training with proper form. It's especially important to maintain proper form when you're training your legs because of the potential for knee or back strain. Never sacrifice form for the amount of weight that you are lifting, and take your time between sets.

During each exercise, bring your navel toward your spine by flexing your lower-abdominal muscles. Move slowly on each repetition—three seconds up, three seconds down. Breathe normally unless you prefer to exhale during the exertion phase. If your legs are still sore from a previous workout, take the day off or do some easy activity. If you feel a twinge of pain on any exercise, stop immediately and seek the advice of your physician.

YOUR PERSONAL TRAINER

Train both your fast- and slow-twitch thigh and bun muscles in the same week by doing 10 to 12 reps in one workout with lighter weights, and doing 6 to 8 reps on your next workout with heavier weights.

Roman Chair Hip Extension

The Roman Chair Hip Extension is a great exercise for your buns. You may perform this exercise with a partner or on a leg-curl or hip-extension machine. Be sure you are hinging at the hip and not the waist. Don't move your upper body too far in either direction. Only go down a few inches below parallel and then come back up a few inches past the parallel position. Place your arms across your chest.

If this exercise is too challenging, use your arms to help press your body into the up position. Take your time—three seconds up and three seconds down works great. If that's too difficult, one second up and one second down is fine as long as your range of motion is only an inch or so.

If placing your arms across your chest is not challenging enough, interlock your fingers behind your head. Breathe normally throughout the entire range of motion of this exercise. If you have back problems, choose a different exercise. You can add a weight across your chest to increase the intensity of the exercise.

1. Place the backs of your ankles underneath the foot pad; your hips should straddle the pad in front.

2. Place your arms across your chest and allow gravity to let your body descend.

3. Flex your buns and raise your upper body back up to a parallel position.

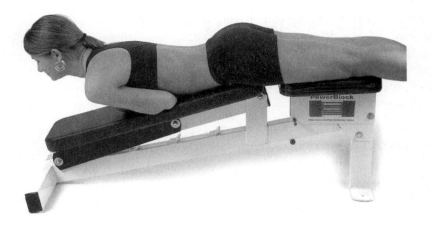

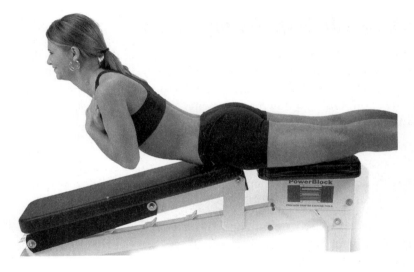

Stiff-Legged Dead Lifts

Stiff-Legged Dead Lifts are one of the best exercises you can do to firm your buns and hamstrings. Use very light weight or no weight at all when beginning this routine. Be sure your back doesn't round out. Press through your heels to target your buns and hamstrings. Consciously focus on flexing your buns and hamstrings.

You must keep your back straight, chest out, stomach in, and shoulders back when you do this exercise. Visualize a steel rod that goes up your back to help keep proper form on this exercise. Breathe normally or, if you prefer, you may exhale during the up phase of this lift. If you're currently suffering from back pain, do a different exercise instead. Try the Lying on Your Stomach Buns Blaster exercise from Chapter 16. This exercise firms your buns and strengthens your back. Be sure to get your doctor's approval before trying it.

1. Stand with your feet a little less than shoulder-width apart, knees slightly bent, and grab the weights with an overhand grip.

2. Slowly descend until you feel a light stretch in your hamstrings and buns. Keep the weights as close to your legs as possible.

3. Flex your buns and hamstrings and move back to your original position.

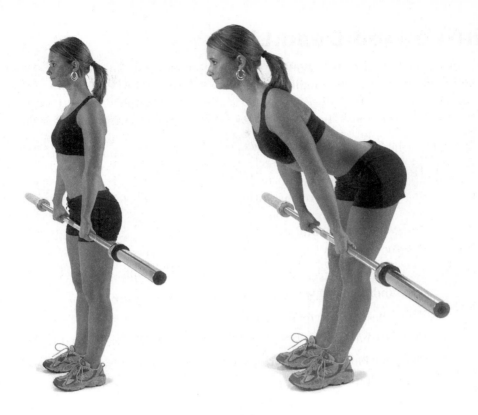

Good-Mornings

Good-Mornings train your buns and hamstrings. At first, use very light weight or no weight at all. As you progress, gradually increase weight, but not at the expense of perfect form. You must keep your back straight, head up, and shoulders back when you perform this exercise. Keep your head level and don't raise it up as you lean forward; this will reduce strain during the exercise. Press through your heels and keep both knees slightly bent. Consciously focus on flexing your buns and hamstrings. If you're currently suffering from back pain, do a different exercise, such as the hip extension explained next.

BET YOU DIDN'T KNOW

Training your legs with weights is a full-body exercise because many muscles in your upper body are used to stabilize your movement.

1. Stand with your feet a little less than shoulder-width apart, knees slightly bent, and hold the weight on the back of your shoulders.

2. Flex your buns and hamstrings as you hinge from the hip and lean forward a few inches.

3. Move back to your original position.

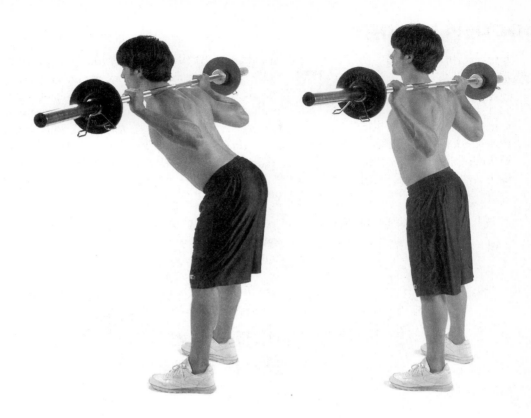

Hip Extension

The Hip Extension tones your buns and hamstrings. Use very light weight to begin with. When you can perform 10 reps with perfect form, add weight. Move three seconds up and three seconds down. If that is too difficult, one second up and one second down is fine.

At first, alternate legs. As you become stronger, you may perform all of your sets with one leg before switching to the other leg. Eventually you may perform this exercise lifting both legs simultaneously. Breathe normally or, if you prefer, exhale on the up phase. Be careful not to lift your legs more than an inch or two.

1. Lie on your stomach and place your arms by your sides. Attach the weights to the backs of your ankles. Lift your right leg 3 inches off of the floor, hinging from the hip. Switch legs and repeat.

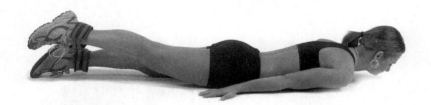

One-Legged Quarter-Squat with Dumbbells

The One-Legged Quarter-Squat with Dumbbells firms up your thighs, buns, hamstrings, and inner/outer thighs. You're working the legs in front when you perform this exercise. Be sure not to bend farther than a 90-degree angle with your front knee. Press through your heel to target the back of your legs and buns. Breathe normally or exhale on the up phase if you prefer. Begin with very light weight. It is advisable to have a wall next to you for balance.

GET IT RIGHT

Keeping your back straight really means maintaining a natural curve in your lower back. This keeps your spinal disks healthy and prevents injury.

1. Begin in a lunge position with your right foot forward and a dumbbell in each hand.

2. Extend your right leg pushing from your heel. Your left leg is there for the purpose of balance only.

3. Switch legs and repeat.

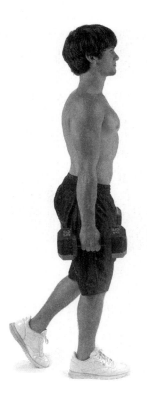
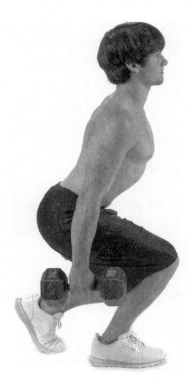

Step-Ups with a Bench

Step-Ups with a Bench work your thighs, buns, hamstrings, and inner/outer thighs. Choose a low bench and maintain your balance throughout the exercise. Your bench should be low enough that you do not shift your body weight using momentum.

Breathe normally or, if you prefer, exhale during the up phase. You should be able to hold your position at any point during your repetition. Maintain perfect posture and resist the urge to lean too far forward as you step up. Press through your heels to train the backs of your legs or press through the balls of your feet to focus on your thighs.

1. Stand in front of a low bench with a dumbbell in each hand.

2. Step onto the bench with your right foot and let your left foot swing naturally so that you are standing on the bench with both feet. Step down with your right foot and then step down with your left foot.

3. Step onto the bench with your left foot and let your right foot swing naturally so that you are standing on the bench with both feet. Step down with your left foot and then step down with your right foot.

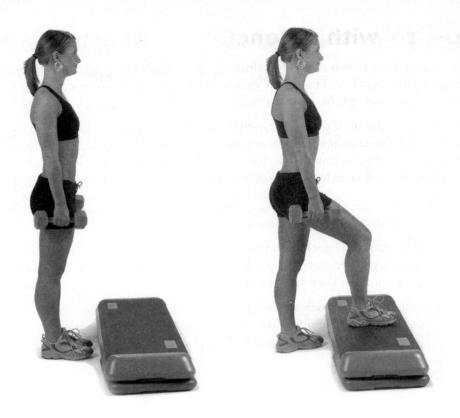

Single-Legged Squat with a Bench

The Single-Legged Squat with a Bench works your thighs, buns, hamstrings, and inner and outer thighs. It requires strength, flexibility, and balance—that's why this is such a great exercise!

Try this exercise without weight. At first, alternate legs. When you feel strong enough, try 10 repetitions with one leg and then switch to the other. When you can successfully perform 10 repetitions with perfect form with either leg, hold a light dumbbell in each hand. Move as slowly as you can for the duration of this exercise.

1. Stand with your left foot on a low bench and your right foot on the floor. Hold a set of dumbbells in each hand.

2. Press your left heel into the bench to raise your body up until your right foot taps the bench. Don't lock your knee out when you rise from the squat.

3. Lower yourself slowly to the floor and complete 10 repetitions.

4. Switch legs and repeat.

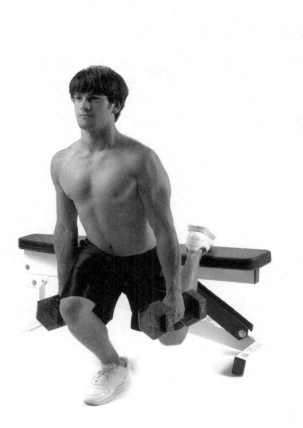

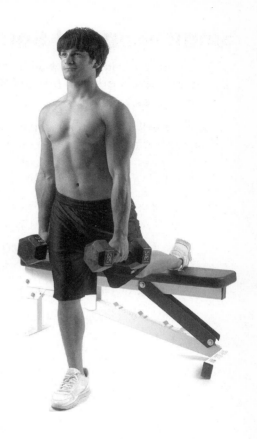

The Least You Need to Know

- Start with lighter weights to get the feel of an exercise and secure proper form before progressing to heavier ones.
- Keep your back straight, stomach in, chest out, and eyes forward.
- Stiff-Legged Dead Lifts are an excellent exercise to firm your buns and hamstrings.

Stretch and Burn

In This Chapter

- Melt fat from your hips and thighs
- Variety keeps you coming back
- Stretch and tone buns and thighs

Losing the fat that surrounds your buns and thighs is easier than you may think. It's not about working in your "target heart rate range." The way to melt fat is simply to move. Did you know that you could burn up to 600 calories a day just by fidgeting? This chapter shows you how to accelerate fat loss doing your favorite activities and stretches that will keep your lower body flexible and ready to move.

Showtime Squats

Watching TV doesn't have to be a sedentary activity. Just doing a minute or two of squats and lunges during the commercials will have you huffing and puffing. Maintain perfect form and alternate 10 reps of squats and 10 reps of lunges with each leg. Move through that cycle until the commercials are over. You will be glad there is a long break until your next set. March in place between squats to reinvigorate your legs. You can also dance around, jump rope, do jumping jacks, walk, march, or run in place. The fat surrounding your hips doesn't know the difference between activities.

BET YOU DIDN'T KNOW

You may do easy activity and cardio every day. But weight training should be limited to twice a week per muscle group.

The harder you work, the sooner your buns and thighs will take shape. If you do 100 squats during a two-minute commercial break, you won't be able to get off the couch for the next commercial. But remember, results don't show from just one workout, so make it a habit every time you watch TV.

Working Your Way Up

If you're overweight and have not worked out since high school or for a long time, and you have the good fortune to belong to a gym, begin on a recumbent bicycle. The recumbent bike allows you to lean back to support your body weight. This requires you to work only against the resistance of the bike without having to support your body weight.

Breathing is also easier for some people on a recumbent. Because your legs are up higher than a normal stationary bike, and they are pedaling horizontally, there is less stress to your cardiovascular system. Recumbent bikes are also great for people who've had previous knee injuries.

YOUR PERSONAL TRAINER

Breathe from your belly (diaphragm). You can get more air into your lungs if you belly breathe.

After you have mastered the recumbent bicycle, move to upright cycling. Upright cycling is more demanding, but it still supports your body weight.

Treadmill walking at an easy pace without an incline is your next step. After you have mastered treadmill walking at an easy pace with no incline, increase the grade to 1 percent. Walking at a 1 percent grade is challenging. But your body will adapt. When it does, increase your pace.

Your next step is the stair-stepping machine. (These machines are also called stepmills.) This vertical movement pattern burns more calories and is very challenging, so be patient with your progress.

After stair stepping comes stair climbing. Stair-climbing machines require even greater effort because you are lifting your body weight repeatedly.

Stair climbing is the final step in your progress up the fat-burning machines at the gym. When you get to stair climbing, work on different speed intervals to challenge yourself.

How soon you move from one exercise device to the next depends on you. An average progression is several weeks on each piece of equipment before moving up.

Remember that cross-training keeps you fresh. Try pedaling one day and climbing stairs the next. On the treadmill, change the pace depending on how you feel. Go fast on a good day. If you don't feel like working out, warm up and then enjoy an easy stroll. Variety is the key to preventing boredom during your workouts.

Whether you use a treadmill, stair climber, elliptical machine, ski machine, or stationary bike, choose an activity that you love that keeps you moving. All of these devices are useful for firming and sculpting your thighs and buns.

But if walking on a treadmill makes you feel like a gerbil, and pedaling on a stationary bike gets you nowhere, do household chores. Vacuuming, sweeping, mopping, or washing windows burns fat and tones those thighs and buns. Your legs are your foundation for every movement you make. Next time you're loading the dishwasher, notice that the muscles in your legs are flexed. You are firming and toning without knowing it.

Walk Before You Jog

Performing lower-body rhythmic activity requires you to use your largest muscle groups in repetitive movements. Begin slowly and progress gradually. Walking for 30 minutes will prepare your muscles for jogging. When you can walk continuously for 30 minutes, you are ready to jog.

On your first walk-jog workout, walk for seven minutes and then jog for three. Jog at a fast walking pace. Repeat this three times for a total of 30 minutes. When you feel ready, walk for five minutes and then jog for five. In a few months you may be able to jog the entire 30 minutes.

> **GET IT RIGHT**
>
> Be careful not to develop an overuse injury. One of the greatest predictors of developing another injury is if you are suffering from a current injury.

Jog in an upright position, stomach in, strike with the heel and then roll to the toe, taking short, smooth strides. Pick up your feet, lifting your front knee, and extending your back leg. Keep your elbows bent, and your forearms and chin parallel to the ground. Breathe deeply from your diaphragm. If you feel winded, slow to a walk. Don't ignore discomfort in your shins, knees, or back. Pay attention to your body.

Stretching Your Buns and Thighs

Have you noticed that on warm days you can touch your toes, but on cooler days you can barely reach your knees? That you can hold your stretch more comfortably in the afternoon than in the morning?

Muscles need to be warm to be able to comfortably stretch. For safety, never stretch a cold muscle. Warm up for five to eight minutes before stretching to avoid injuries. Exhale as you move into each position. Learn to hold your stretch for at least 10 seconds in order to fully relax the muscle. Add 2 seconds a week until you work up to 30 seconds. You may stretch to a slight level of tension, but never approaching pain.

Figure-4 Stretch

The Figure-4 Stretch lengthens your buns and outer thigh muscles. Keep your back straight and your head on the floor. Your neck should remain relaxed. Move slowly through your stretch. Stretch to the point of tension, never discomfort. Relax into your stretch.

After a few months, stretch even farther by using your hands to pull your leg slowly toward your chest. When you feel tension, stop, and then relax.

1. Lie on your back with your legs in a Figure-4 position. Your right ankle is pressed to your left thigh.

2. Slowly draw your left thigh toward your chest.

3. Switch legs and repeat.

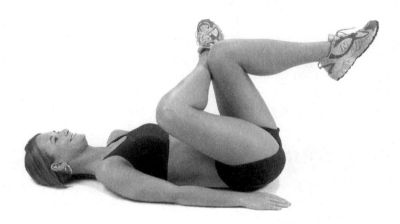

Straddle Stretch

The Straddle Stretch loosens your inner thighs and hamstrings. Lead with your chest, keep your head up, shoulders back, and relax. Walk your hands out in front and focus on your hamstrings and inner thighs. Keep your toes pointed up and do not allow your back to round. Hinge from your hip. Keep your back and knees straight. Exhale into your stretch.

1. Sit with your legs spread out as far as comfortable.

2. Slowly lower your chest toward the floor.

3. When you feel tension, stop and hold.

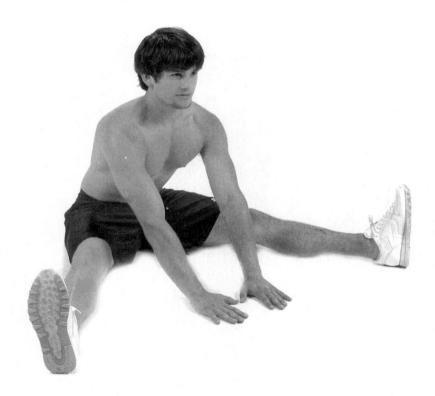

Thigh Stretch

The Thigh Stretch lengthens the front of your upper leg. Maintain perfect posture and relax into the stretch. Resist the temptation to look down at your foot.

After a few months, attempt the stretch without using the wall for balance. A few months after that, if you feel comfortable, grab the top of your foot with your other hand. If you have knee problems, you may choose a different stretch.

1. Stand with your right hand holding a wall for balance. Bend your left knee behind you and grab the top of your left foot with your left hand. Exhale and hold.

2. Switch legs and repeat.

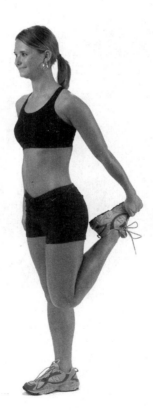

Side of Thigh Stretch

The Side of Thigh Stretch lengthens the muscle and tendon on the side of your upper thigh. Relax into your stretch until you feel light tension. This stretch improves with practice. It doesn't matter how far someone else can stretch, or what the model in the photo does. The more flexible you are, the farther you have to stretch. You may practice this stretch without a wall.

1. Stand with your feet together. Your right hip should be facing the wall. Place your right hand on the wall and lean your right hip toward the wall.

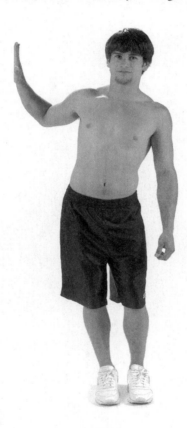

Butt Stretch

The Butt Stretch is very relaxing after sitting all day. Be aware that one hip may be more flexible than the other. Hinge from your hip and keep your back straight. Keep your shoulders down and your neck in line with your spine. Exhale and hold each stretch until you feel tension.

1. Sit with one leg crossed over the other and your knees bent.

2. Lean forward, leading with your chest until you feel a stretch in your buns.

3. Switch legs and repeat.

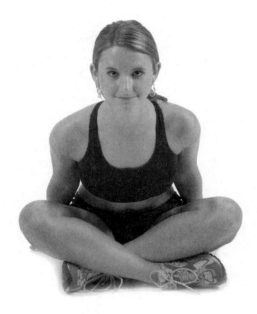

The Least You Need to Know

- Burn fat in your buns and thighs by working your way through different machines at the gym.
- Vary your workout routine to prevent boredom.
- Stretching is most beneficial when the muscles are warm.

Additional Resources

Workouts are constantly changing thanks to new technology, better equipment, and innovative ideas. Keep pace with the latest fitness toys, tools, and news in these great magazines, DVDs/videos, and websites.

Magazines to Motivate Your Upper-Body Workout

Magazines can provide you with the latest buzz on your upper-body training. But be careful. Sometimes the latest information presented in magazines may be tied to a product they are selling in an adjacent ad. But at least you can look at the pictures for inspiration.

Flex

Health

Iron Man Magazine

Men's Health

Muscle and Fitness

Muscle and Fitness Hers

Natural Bodybuilding

Women's Health

Videos to Change Up Your Upper-Body Routine

If you enjoy training to videos and DVDs, go for it. After you learn the movements, adjust the weights and reps to your specific upper-body routine. I hope you enjoy some of these videos. Take away as much information from the videos as possible, regardless of whether the video personality gets on your nerves.

Cory Everson's Get Hard Arms & Shoulders

The Firm: Body Sculpting System 2—Upper Body Sculpt

The Firm: Upper Body Split

Gilad's Quick Fit Chest & Back

Gilad's Quick Fit Shoulders & Arms

Leslie Sansone's Short Cuts Upper Body

Videos and DVDs are available at:

Collage Video
5390 Main Street NE
Minneapolis, MN 55421
800-433-6769
www.collagevideo.com

Magazines to Motivate Your Abs Training

Looking at photos of magazine models with amazing abs may inspire you to get your ab workout in. You may notice that there is nothing new with regard to ab training, but at least you can try some tips if they are substantiated by research.

Men's Health

Muscle and Fitness Hers

Oxygen

Weight Watchers

Women's Health

Yoga Journal

Videos to Change Up Your Abs Routine

There are only so many ways to train your abs. But these videos are particularly informative about training your back as well.

Best Abs on Earth

The Firm: 5-Day Abs

Gilad's Quick Fit Abs

Karen Voight's Core Essentials

Leslie Sansone's Short Cuts Abs

Magazines to Motivate Your Buns and Thigh Training

Fitness

Men's Fitness

Ms. Fitness

Self

Shape

Videos to Change Up Your Buns and Thigh Routine

The Firm: Lower Body Sculpt I

The Firm: Lower Body Split

The Firm: Sculpted Buns, Hips & Thighs

Janis Saffell's Brand New Butt & More

Karen Voight's Lean Legs and Buns

Leslie Sansone's Short Cuts Lower Body

Websites to Bolster Your Total Body Workout

You can find just about anything you need to know in the world of body fitness, from the latest news and techniques to eating programs to virtual coaches. Here are some websites to get you started:

American Council on Exercise
www.acefitness.org

Berkeley Wellness Letter
www.berkeleywellness.com

Calorie Control Council
www.caloriecontrol.org

Cooper Institute
www.cooperaerobics.com

Food and Nutrition Information Center
www.nal.usda.gov/fnic/index.html

Gatorade Sports Science Institute
www.gssiweb.org

IDEA: Health & Fitness Association
www.ideafit.com

NetSweat.com: The Internet's Fitness Resource
www.netsweat.com

NSCA: National Strength and Conditioning Association
www.nsca-lift.org

Nutrition Data
www.nutritiondata.com

Tom Seabourne's website
www.tomseabourne.com

Index

C

N-O

U